HEALING
ANXIETY
with HERBS

OTHER BOOKS BY HAROLD H. BLOOMFIELD, M.D.
(authored and co-authored):

*TM: Discovering Inner Energy and Overcoming
     Stress*
Happiness
Holistic Way to Health and Happiness
How to Enjoy the Love of your Life
How to Heal Depression
How to Survive the Loss of a Love
Hypericum (Saint-John's-wort) *& Depression*
Inner Joy
Lifemates
Love Secrets for a Lasting Relationship
Making Peace in Your Stepfamily
Making Peace with Your Parents
Making Peace with Yourself
*Surviving, Healing and Growing: The How to
     Survive the Loss of a Love Workbook*
The Power of 5
Think Safe, Be Safe

HEALING
ANXIETY
with HERBS

HAROLD H. BLOOMFIELD, M.D.

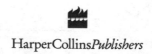

HarperCollins*Publishers*

HarperCollins books may be purchased for educational, business, or sales promotional use. For information please write: Special Markets Department, HarperCollins Publishers, Inc., 10 East 53rd Street, New York, NY 10022.

FIRST EDITION

Designed by Laura Lindgren

Library of Congress Cataloging-in-Publication Data

Bloomfield, Harold H., 1944–
 Healing anxiety with herbs / Harold H. Bloomfield. — 1st ed.
  p. cm.
 Includes bibliographical references and index.
 ISBN 0-06-019127-9
  1. Anxiety—Alternative treatment. 2. Herbs—Therapeutic use.
 I. Title.
 RC531.B56 1998
 616.85'22306—dc21   98-1427

98 99 00 01 02 ❖/RRD 10 9 8 7 6 5 4

This book is dedicated to
the herbal medicines of Mother Nature,
to the beautiful *Blooms* in my *Field*—
Sirah, Shazara, Damien, Michael, Fridl, and Nora,
and to you, dear reader, on your healing journey.

*The Lord hath created medicines out of the earth,
and he that is wise will not abhor them.*
—ECCLESIASTES 38:4

CONTENTS

PART 3
NATURAL SELF-HEALING

IMPORTANT INFORMATION

READ THIS FIRST

This book is not intended to be a guide for self-medication. A reliable diagnosis can only be made by a physician. For this reason professional advice should always be sought before undertaking self-administered herbal therapy. Only in this way can you make safe use of the beneficial effects of herbs.

Healing Anxiety with Herbs is intended to be educational and is in no way a substitute for advice from a physician or mental health professional. Always verify with your doctor the correct dosage before taking any natural remedy described in this book. Never administer any remedy to a child without a physician's advice. Herbs can interact with other drugs you are taking or have adverse effects themselves. If you are currently taking prescription medication for anxiety, please do not change your dosage without medical guidance. If you are taking a prescription tranquilizer, sleeping pill, or antidepressant and suddenly stop, withdrawal symptoms can be severe.

More medical research is necessary to chart the applications, usefulness, and limitations of herbal therapy for anxiety more precisely and reliably. The author and publisher expressly disclaim responsibility for any negative effects directly or indirectly attributable to the use or application of any information contained in this book.

INTRODUCTION

*Vis medicatrix naturae. (Honor the healing power of
nature.)*

—Hippocrates

Anxious? Stressed? Have difficulty calming yourself into a
deep, natural sleep? Well, you are not alone. Over sixty-five
million Americans suffer annually from anxiety, chronic
stress, and insomnia. Until recently the only option for many
was prescription antianxiety and sleeping pills. But these
drugs can bring with them impaired memory, loss of concentration, poor quality of sleep, addiction, and withdrawal
symptoms. Remarkably safe, highly effective herbal medicines
are revolutionizing the treatment of mild to moderate anxiety, depression, and insomnia. These natural remedies are
available without a prescription and are free of the side
effects and addiction potential associated with synthetic
drugs. Mounting scientific evidence, including studies published in the *Journal of the American Medical Association, New
England Journal of Medicine, British Medical Journal,* and other
leading periodicals, is documenting the validity, safety—and
increasing popularity—of herbal medicines.

While herbs have been valued as folk remedies since
ancient times, modern medical science has only recently confirmed their healing properties. Kava, a natural tranquilizer,
does not have the side effects of Valium-like benzodiazepines
(such as Xanax and Klonopin) but can be a more effective

cure for the millions of people with mild to moderate anxiety. *Hypericum* (Saint-John's-wort), which can be just as effective as synthetic antidepressants for depression, can also help reduce anxiety and maintain emotional harmony. Valerian, a natural herbal sedative, can provide a good night's sleep without the morning hangover or rebound insomnia of prescription sleeping pills such as Dalmane, Halcion, and Restoril. *Ginkgo biloba* is a brain booster that should be considered as a daily supplement by anyone over the age of forty dealing with the angst of aging. Adaptogenic herbs, like ginseng, eleuthero, and ashwaganda, can help strengthen the nervous system and protect against stress. Aromatherapy is being used in Europe to calm patients before surgery and in the treatment of attention deficit disorder.

Healing Anxiety with Herbs provides specific information that will allow you, in consultation with your health care professional, to make an informed choice about whether you need treatment for anxiety and how herbal medicines can be used for healing. Herbal remedies are only appropriate for mild to moderate anxiety, not severe cases. Synthetic drugs are necessary and helpful for major anxiety disorders. I still write prescriptions, but, as I can attest, natural healing is best.

I have wanted to be a physician and psychiatrist ever since I can remember. I identify proudly with the great Greek physician Hippocrates (460–377 B.C.), the father of medicine, who regularly prescribed herbal medicines for "nervous unrest." So it is a great sadness for me to point out a tragic flaw in modern medicine's treatment of anxiety. Pharmaceutical companies warn, in the drug packaging inserts for benzodiazepine tranquilizers (Xanax, Valium, Klonopin, and Ativan) and sleeping pills (Restoril, Dalmane, Serax, and Halcion) that these drugs are not to be used for longer than three weeks, because they rapidly become addictive. Often they create rebound anxiety and insomnia when withdrawn. Yet many physicians routinely renew these prescriptions for months and even years. Millions of people have become addicted to these legal prescription drugs, more than the total number who abuse heroin and cocaine. Hundreds of thousands of people suffer from memory loss, poor concentration, and imbalance as side effects of these drugs, resulting in tens of thousands of automobile accidents, hip fractures from falls, and unnecessary deaths.

Every day I get heart-wrenching phone calls from patients who have suffered physically, emotionally, and financially from doctors relentlessly pushing these drugs upon them. These patients have frequently been told that they have no other choice but to continue to take benzodiazepines over the long term. They bitterly complain that their doctors just write prescriptions and don't suggest any means by which patients can help themselves. When patients inquire if their anxiety can be treated with herbal medicines, they are often met with cynicism. In medical offices and clinics, millions of people are crippled annually, not by their anxiety but by a reflexive "take-this-prescription" mentality. This further disempowers the anxious person and can interfere with true healing.

The physician is only nature's assistant.

—Galen

What compounds these human tragedies is that they are avoidable. Europeans already use herbal tranquilizers and sleep aids more frequently than prescription drugs. America is significantly behind Germany, France, and England in the use of herbal medicines to heal anxiety, because of a lack of information in America about their proven medical effectiveness. Whereas German physicians are trained in the use of herbs during medical school, and over three-fourths of German doctors prescribe them in their practice, most American physicians continue to write prescriptions for tranquilizers and sleeping pills routinely, without knowledge of these safer natural alternatives.

Antianxiety drugs are a multibillion-dollar business. The pharmaceutical industry helps underwrite medical journals, professional meetings, and drug representatives who bring free samples to doctors' offices. While there is a huge profit incentive for developing and testing a new synthetic tranquilizer or antidepressant drug, there is no economic incentive for U.S. companies to research an herbal medicine alternative, because a plant remedy cannot be patented.

The growing popularity of herbs has been primarily a consumer-led revolution. The new field of *phytomedicine* (plant medicine) subjects herbal remedies to the same exacting research standards that modern science uses for synthetic drugs—double-blind, placebo-controlled studies at major medical centers. Consequently, medicinal herbs for anxiety have received scientific validation in both clinical and laboratory studies. As the effectiveness of plant medicines becomes more widely known, there will surely be greater acceptance by U.S. health professionals and the general public.

For the tens of millions of Americans who suffer from mild to moderate anxiety, chronic stress, and insomnia, rational medicine would dictate that herbs be considered as a first-line treatment. Doctor and patient should only proceed to more powerful (and dangerous) prescription tranquilizers and sleeping pills if an adequate course of natural remedies fails. More American physicians than ever are recommending herbal medicines, but unfortunately they are still in the minority. The federal government has begun vitally needed

U.S. research studies through the Office of Alternative Medicine at the National Institutes of Health. This federal agency, established in 1993, is giving grants to leading medical institutions to study the efficacy of Hypericum and other herbs for the treatment of depression, anxiety, and other conditions.

The goal of this guide is to be practical, accurate, and compassionate. The last thing you want when you're feeling anxious is a thick tome weighed down with footnotes, long citations, Latin terms, and impenetrable jargon. Anxiety and depression cause suffering; I know because I've been there. *Healing Anxiety with Herbs* is divided into three sections.

PART 1: WHAT IS ANXIETY?

Some anxiety is normal, serving to protect you from real danger and to stimulate change and growth. Anxiety becomes maladaptive when you react to situations that do not pose a real threat. This section explores the basic questions about anxiety: What causes anxiety? How does one become anxious? What are the signs and symptoms? What are the most common types? How is anxiety healed? When is treatment necessary? How are stress and anxiety related? When does stress endanger one's health?

PART 2: HERBS FOR ANXIETY, INSOMNIA, AND STRESS

Herbal medicines are revolutionizing the treatment of anxiety. Kava, made from the root of a Polynesian pepper tree, could replace Valium, Xanax, and other tranquilizers for relief of mild to moderate anxiety. Medical studies have shown that kava can often relieve mild to moderate anxiety as effectively as benzodiazepine tranquilizers but with no sedation, memory impairment, or significant threat of addiction.

Valerian, an East Indian root, is sometimes called nature's Valium. It has been medically proven to reduce the amount of time it takes to fall asleep and to improve sleep quality. Unlike Restoril, Dalmane, Halcion, and other commonly prescribed sleeping pills, valerian is not addictive and has been safely used as a sleep aid for centuries. In Europe a doctor is likely first to recommend valerian for insomnia and to prescribe a sleeping pill only in a smaller number of cases where a stronger drug may be briefly needed.

> *Medicus curat, natura sanat. (Medicine treats, nature heals.)*
>
> —Ambroise Paré, the father
> of modern surgery

You will learn about the antistress and antifatigue herbs— *Panax* ginseng, Siberian ginseng, ashwaganda, and licorice root—that act as nerve tonics (i.e., they can strengthen the nervous system). Sedative herbs, such as California poppy, Reishi mushroom, and chamomile, can help you stay calm and relaxed so that you don't feel the need for a tranquilizer. Many people over the age of forty should consider taking *Ginkgo biloba* to protect the brain and milk thistle to protect the liver. Exciting new research on herbal medicines from China, Japan, India, and South America will be explored. For example, hospitals in Britain are using lavender and other aromatherapy herbal scents to enhance patients' recovery. Evening primrose oil and traditional Chinese medicinal herbs are being used in the treatment of attention deficit disorder.

PART 3: NATURAL SELF-HEALING

*The doctor of the future will give no medicine, but will
interest his patients in the care of the human frame, in
diet, and in the cause and prevention of disease.*
                                        —Thomas Edison

Although herbal medicines can be effective on their own,
they work best when they are part of a natural self-healing
program. Research suggests that healing anxiety is innate
and natural, but anxiety also signals a need to change to a
more healthful, natural lifestyle. Ultraspecific, highly practical, natural self-healing tools and strategies can be used on
the spot, wherever you are, so that you feel less like a *human
doing* and more like a *human being*. In this natural self-healing
program you will learn specific exercises to:

- Become more at ease and revitalize your mind and body
  in the midst of a hectic schedule
- Sleep more soundly, night after night
- Overcome fear to accomplish more of your goals and
  ambitions
- Maintain lifelong health and emotional fitness without
  strain or hassles
- Create genuine inner peace and pleasure
- Decrease unnecessary worry
- Express what you really feel and want
- Make anger work for you
- Boost your spirit to bring out more of your best during
  stressful times
- Effectively deal with the anxiety of loss and change dur-
  ing the three stages of healing
- Resolve a spiritual crisis and renew your soul

Nature is made to conspire with spirit to emancipate us.
                                    —Ralph Waldo Emerson

    Botanical medicines tap the creative intelligence of nature to heal our nervous system. Herbal remedies and natural self-healing can help us to transcend our separation anxiety and become whole again. By attunement to the natural, herbal medicines allow us to rediscover the "lost paradise," not in some nether world or mystical state but right here on earth. While modern pharmaceuticals will always be important for severe disorders, herbal extracts have a major, vital role to play in healing the mild to moderate anxiety that so many of us suffer from every day. Synthetic drugs are certainly valuable when necessary, but the power of herbal medicines has been underrecognized and underutilized. Natural remedies can be truly transformative in their healing ability. I am hopeful that this book will make an important contribution to your life and to healing anxiety in America.

PART I

WHAT IS ANXIETY?

There is no question that the problem of anxiety is a nodal point at which the most various and important questions converge, a riddle whose solution would be bound to throw a flood of light on our whole mental existence.

—SIGMUND FREUD

1

You Are Not Alone

The only thing we have to fear is fear itself—nameless, unreasoning, unjustified terror which paralyses needed efforts to convert retreat into advance.
—FRANKLIN D. ROOSEVELT

All human beings experience fear, a necessary signal of real danger. As children, most of us had fears of the dark. The fear of physical pain and emotional suffering is a natural part of being alive. When the word *anxiety* is used in this book, it refers to mild to moderate anxiety, not to an anxiety disorder. Herbs are most useful for mild to moderate anxiety.

Feelings of anxiety come in many forms: alarm, anguish, dread, anger, fright, horror, panic, and terror. Physical complaints can include jumpiness, racing heart rate, trembling, cold and/or clammy hands, dizziness, upset stomach, diarrhea, flush, faintness, rapid breathing, numbness, tingling, strain, and fatigue. Anxiety can strike like lightning or rumble, ever present, in the background. It can be the natural fear that accompanies life's challenges and major difficulties (e.g., losing a job or becoming seriously ill). It can also be marked by chronic edginess and worry. The feelings and physical sensations of anxiety are the same whether it occurs spontaneously or in direct response to a major threat.

Anxiety is an overreaction in the first stage of the body's stress response, the alarm ("fight or flight") reaction. Mild to moderate anxiety, in particular, may be a more exaggerated and intense stress response. Remember, if you suffer from inappropriate fears or persistent worrying, you are not alone. Research has shown that:

- Each year sixty-five million Americans experience some symptoms of anxiety, of whom thirty million have a full-blown disorder. Medicine uses terms like *subclinical, syndromal, minor,* and *shadow syndromes* to describe the mild to moderate anxiety of the thirty-five million people whose symptoms are not severe or numerous enough to qualify as an anxiety disorder. One of every two people will experience mild to moderate anxiety for at least a two-week period during their lifetime; one of four people will suffer from an anxiety disorder.
- Anxiety in its various forms—worry, insomnia, heart palpitations, muscle aches and pains, rapid shallow breathing, nausea, headaches, fatigue—is one of the more common complaints heard by doctors. Anxiety can provoke or worsen overeating, alcoholism, premenstrual syndrome, irritable bowel syndrome, and other medical problems.
- Despite the fact that more people suffer from anxiety than any other mental health problem, less than 25 percent receive adequate help. This means that some eighteen million people continue to suffer unnecessarily from a treatable condition.
- More than twice as many women suffer from anxiety as men. It is not known whether this is because women are more likely to be anxious or because men are more likely

to deny being afraid. Men are more likely than women to turn to alcohol and drug abuse to mask their anxiety.

- According to a 1997 Gallup poll, as much as 25 percent of the U.S. workforce suffers from anxiety and chronic stress, which it is estimated costs U.S. businesses sixty to seventy-five billion dollars a year.

ANXIETY CHECK

Do you experience anxiety? We all do in some form or another, but the question is how much and how often. The quizzes below will help you determine the degree to which you suffer from anxiety. These self-assessments are also a way of measuring your progress as you heal. You should consult your physician or a trained mental health professional to diagnose your anxiety accurately and appropriately.

The measurement of anxiety has height and width—the degree of anxiety you are experiencing and the frequency with which you experience it. When you can recognize and label the symptoms of anxiety, they often become less frightening. Remember the dictum, "When you label me, you negate me." These quizzes are a measurement of your anxiety level, not of you. You are a magnificent being, much more than the momentary quantifying of the "noise" or "static" in your nervous system.

Remember that while herbal treatments are best for mild to moderate anxiety, even severe anxiety is highly treatable with psychiatric medications, and as your symptoms lessen, herbs can be used. Also, you will learn a potent natural self-healing program of emotional fitness, stress reduction, exercise, nutrition, vitamins, and supplements that can help heal any level of anxiety and maintain your well-being.

QUIZ 1: SITUATIONAL ANXIETY

For each situation below, indicate the degree of anxiety you experience on a scale from 0 to 3:

    0 = no anxiety

    1 = mild anxiety

    2 = moderate anxiety

    3 = severe anxiety

Situations that might elicit anxiety, fear, or tension:
- Coming home to an empty house
- Going to sleep or waking up
- Going to a doctor or dentist
- Driving a car
- Taking a plane flight
- Entering an elevator
- Being in a crowd
- The thought of death
- Taking a business call
- Making a major purchase or investment
- Speaking to a group
- Eating alone in a restaurant
- Being in enclosed places
- Waiting in line
- Packing for a trip
- Making "cold calls" at work
- Giving or receiving a gift
- Socializing at a party
- The sight of blood
- Talking to people in authority
- Being criticized
- Going to a public restroom
- Feeling stared at
- Confronting a loved one about a problem

- Financial obligations, unpaid bills
- Deadlines, evaluations, or tests
- Heavy commuter traffic
- Being on time for appointments or events
- Keeping things neat and orderly
- Sexual performance
- Being seen naked or in a bathing suit
- Making a mistake, failing
- Rejection in love or at work

Scoring
20 to 39 = mild to moderate anxiety
40 to 59 = moderate anxiety
60 and over = a possible anxiety disorder

QUIZ 2: SYMPTOMS OF ANXIETY

Indicate the frequency with which you experience each of the following physical and mental symptoms on a scale from 0 to 3:
    0 = never
    1 = mild frequency; a little bit
    2 = moderate frequency
    3 = very much; almost all the time
    Physical and mental symptoms:
- Nervousness or tension
- Dizziness or faintness
- Trembling or shaking
- Sweating
- Chest pain or tightness
- Rapid heartbeat
- Choking or lump in the throat
- Nausea or abdominal discomfort
- Hyperventilation or difficulty breathing
- Panic

- Frozen smile or tight facial muscles
- Neckaches or backaches
- Numbness of the lips, fingers, or toes
- Irritable bowel or indigestion
- Difficulty sleeping or insomnia
- Odd, sharp pains
- Overeating
- Muscle spasms and weakness
- Feeling unsafe
- Fear of impending doom
- Preoccupation with illness
- Fear of going crazy
- Feeling of being out of control
- Fear of embarrassment or humiliation
- Fear of rejection or disapproval
- Struggle with time, impatience
- Rumination over details
- Guilt-filled memories
- Preoccupation with dirt or germs
- Worry about neatness
- Fear of being ugly or fat
- Questioning of failures and "what-ifs"
- Alcohol and drug abuse

Scoring
20 to 39 = mild to moderate anxiety
40 to 59 = moderate anxiety
60 and over = a possible anxiety disorder

2

"I'm Afraid to Get Help!"

> *No Grand Inquisitor has in readiness such terrible tortures as has anxiety, and no spy knows how to attack more artfully the man he suspects, choosing the instant when he is weakest, nor knows how to lay traps where he will be caught and ensnared, as anxiety knows how.*
>
> —SØREN KIERKEGAARD

Despite the fact that there are effective treatments for anxiety, many of those afflicted never seek help. The common feelings people with anxiety have are "I'm too scared to try anything new," "Why bother?" and "Nothing works"—attitudes that can interfere with reaching out for assistance. The thought of treatment may frighten you initially and appear to add to the worries you already have. While you may be understandably apprehensive about seeking help, effective treatment for anxiety will lighten your load and ease your distress. If you are too scared to drive to a doctor's office on your own, ask a friend or relative to take you. Although seeing a psychia-

trist or psychologist might seem intimidating, a health professional will understand your problems. If you decide to try the
herbal approach, an open-minded psychiatrist, holistic M.D.,
D.O. (osteopathic physician), chiropractor, or N.D. (naturopathic physician) would be preferable (see Appendix C).

Most people respond to antianxiety treatment rapidly,
usually in a matter of days. You may not feel better overnight,
but the sense of being overwhelmed and overburdened should
ease significantly in a short time. Long-term, expensive treatments are seldom necessary. Treatment for anxiety with herbs
is relatively inexpensive. But no matter what the cost, it is
more than compensated for by improved health, greater productivity, and a more satisfying life.

People with anxiety are often afraid of taking medication
because of the fear of side effects. Please note that when compared to synthetic drugs, herbs are much more gentle, freer
of side effects, and nonaddictive.

Don't put off the decision to seek treatment. Two hall-
marks of anxiety are procrastination and indecision. To avoid
"the paralysis of analysis," take immediate constructive
action. Pick up the phone right now to make an appointment
for a consultation. It's important to remember that when you
are anxious, everything and everyone can appear frightening.
You may feel foolish or embarrassed about your obsessions or
phobias. Even seeking help can feel dangerous when perceived through the lens of fear. If you suffer from anxiety, the
only major decision to be made is to get proper diagnosis and
treatment. Other major decisions can wait until your appre-
hensions begin to heal. You won't know how much you can
be helped until you try.

Without treatment, anxiety can worsen. It may progressively interfere with work, family, and almost all other
aspects of life. Left untreated it can last for years, decades, or
a lifetime. Anxiety, in fact, can become so much a "ground of

being" that it's hard to imagine another way of thinking, feeling, or behaving. Persistent anxiety can trigger the onset of disease. Constant worry can increase the risk of a heart attack, precipitate an asthma attack, worsen diabetes, and even increase the risk of cancer. Repeated bouts of anxiety also increase vulnerability to viral infections such as colds, the flu, and herpes.

As long as people consider their anxiety an incorrigible part of their being, they are unlikely to seek diagnosis and treatment. They stay stuck in denial and think, "That's just the way I am." The major problem with anxiety, therefore, is undertreatment. Many people postpone treatment hoping that anxiety will simply go away. This may or may not happen. Treatment for anxiety tends to be more successful the earlier it is begun. And most importantly, the earlier anxiety is treated, the sooner the suffering ends. Remember, procrastinating may be a symptom of anxiety, so don't postpone your healing.

THE FEAR OF GOING CRAZY

*It's not the large things that send a man to the madhouse
. . . not the death of his love but a shoelace that snaps
with no time left.*

—"THE SHOELACE,"
A POEM BY CHARLES BUKOWSKI

Many people try really hard to be what they think is normal, and that is being neurotic. Many of those suffering from anxiety are afraid they are going crazy and try to hide it by staying isolated. A panic attack may be so terrifying that they live in dread of another. Victims later say, "I was sure I was losing my mind or going crazy."

Anxiety disorder is not psychosis. Symptoms of anxiety can sometimes include intrusive or "crazy" thoughts. The fear of going crazy, however, is very different from actual insanity. People with anxiety disorder are *not* more prone to schizophrenia. If in doubt, it is best to get a mental health expert to make a diagnosis. People with anxiety are sometimes secretly ashamed of repeated sexual or aggressive thoughts, especially toward those they love. But there is no symptom of anxiety, no matter how bizarre or repulsive it may appear to you, that has not been experienced by millions of others.

To those who may have anxiety that is due to a psychotic disturbance, do not despair. A psychiatrist is the most appropriate health professional to make the diagnosis between anxiety disorder and schizophrenia. While herbs are not appropriate, modern psychiatric medicines can effectively treat a psychotic disturbance. Phenothiazines and other major tranquilizers have proven very valuable in the treatment of schizophrenia; antidepressant medications have helped those suffering from severe depression; and lithium carbonate or Depakote (divalproex) can alleviate manic-depressive illness.

IF YOU ARE SUICIDAL OR IN A PANIC, GET HELP AT ONCE

If you're afraid that you might act on a suicidal impulse, please call 911 immediately or go to your local hospital emergency room. You should also seek help at once if you:

- Feel in a panic with no one to turn to
- Fear a heart attack or have difficulty breathing
- Feel you are losing control or going crazy (i.e., having a mental breakdown)
- Use excessive amounts of alcohol or abuse drugs

It is common for severely anxious people to have thoughts of suicide. Anxiety is painful, and the mind explores ways to flee from it. For obvious reasons, however, it is important not to *act* upon suicidal feelings. As anxiety heals your outlook, life will improve. Yes, life will still have its ups and downs, and you will feel your fair share of fear, worry, and all the other anxious emotions, but suicide will seldom seem like a solution. Please also see Appendix D for a listing of organizations to call for referrals. This is not the time to be brave and attempt to go it alone. The first step in overcoming anxiety is often the most difficult: finding the courage to ask for help.

FAITH AND FEAR

When I said, "My foot is slipping," your love, O Lord, supported me. When anxiety was great, within me, your consolation brought joy to my soul.

—PSALMS 94:18–19

As powerful as faith in God can be, fear biologically interferes with the brain's ability to trust—to "let go and let God." Like the farmer who casts seeds upon rocks, all the faith and hope in the world may not take hold when presented to a dread-filled mind.

There are two fundamental misconceptions concerning God and anxiety. The first is that suffering is good for you; if you suffer enough, God will be pleased. The martyr is expected to persevere over all anxiety and suffering as a test of faith. The second is that the dread and despair of anxiety are strictly a spiritual test; the only treatment should be God's personal intervention and grace gained through more intense faith and prayer. In fact, God's benevolence comes in many forms and manifests itself in many ways. Among these are herbs from the earth and medical treatments for anxiety. People treated for anxiety find that their faith, spirituality, and trust in a higher power are strengthened. Herbal medicines are truly a gift from God.

Modern medicine prescribes synthetically derived pharmaceuticals as the number one cure. The herbal mind-set more humbly emphasizes that botanicals act as the best catalysts of natural healing. Faith in natural remedies seems to maximize the effectiveness of herbal medicines. From a scientific vantage point, this power of belief, referred to as the placebo effect, is sometimes denigrated, but from a more holistic point of view, faith in herbal medicines is viewed as putting your trust in nature. Indeed, both modern and folk medicines work best when the patient has faith in the remedies and is hopeful of recovery.

Herbal medicines, it should be emphasized, are not placebos. Indeed, placebo-controlled, double-blind medical research is proving that their effectiveness is significantly more than a placebo effect. In these rigorously designed scientific studies, neither the doctors nor their patients know who has been given a placebo or the herbal medicine being tested until the end of the study (hence *double-blind*). In medical research the placebo effect—the power of belief—is considered a distraction that interferes with the study of the actual benefits of the drug or herb. That is why randomly assigned double-blind, placebo-controlled experiments have become the gold standard of research.

The placebo effect, however, is also a testament to the power of faith. Studies of placebo treatments for dozens of ailments, including anxiety disorders, have found that about one-third of patients experience satisfactory relief with a placebo. These placebo-induced cures are not just imaginary or purely subjective but are often the result of real, measurable physiological changes. The placebo effect may be initiated in part by *endorphins*, which are naturally occurring opiate-like hormones in the brain. These biochemical substances are also stimulated, for example, by aerobic exercise and acupuncture. Endorphins reduce the sensation of pain and affect emotions.

Integrative psychiatry emphasizes that an anxious person is not just a passive, helpless spectator in the healing process. Anxious people often suffer from self-doubt; they doubt their own power to heal themselves. The treating physician who just hands the patient a prescription for tranquilizers is conveying more faith in the power of drugs than in the patient's innate healing powers.

Unfortunately, many people who suffer from anxiety are prone to another powerful element of faith, the *Pygmalion effect*, or a tendency to conform to the expectations of an authority figure, such as a doctor. If a physician makes a brusque diagnosis of anxiety, one's health can be negatively influenced. Negative beliefs about your healing too often become self-fulfilling prophecies. On the other hand, if the health care professional shows faith in your natural healing capacity, you are further empowered by the suggestion of herbal medicines and other therapeutic modalities.

The confidence generated by a strong doctor-patient relationship is both a requirement for and a product of natural self-healing. A 1997 study by D. H. Novack *et al.* in the *Journal of the American Medical Association* scientifically demonstrated that the physician has a profound impact on the healing process. A doctor's attitudes, biases, and beliefs are communicated to the patient overtly and covertly. The health care provider's genuine compassion, positive regard, and enthusiasm ("en-theos," to be filled with spirit) is an integral aspect of patient recovery. The word *heal* comes from the old English word *healen*, which means to make whole.

3

Anxiety Alters Relationships

What is stopping you, this very moment, from being the person you want to be and living your life the way you want to live it? The answer—beneath all the other answers—is fear.

—SUSAN JEFFERS, PH.D.,
FEEL THE FEAR AND DO IT ANYWAY

A common symptom of anxiety is a fear of failure or inadequacy. Yet anxiety is a disorder that you can't hold against yourself as a lack of will or understanding. You have nothing to blame yourself for and nothing to feel guilty about. It's hard enough feeling frightened without beating yourself up for it.

People with persistent fear often feel shame, inadequacy, and guilt. They are mercilessly tormented by the fear of fear (i.e., dread of having another panic attack). They may be so easily intimidated that they often become shy and emotionally withdrawn. They can seldom experience the feelings associated with anxiety—fear, anguish, or worry—without looking for a cause. Those who look inside themselves for the cause of their terror may become hypochondriacal or self-absorbed in suffering. Those who look outside tend to feel victimized by their marriage, job, or other life circumstances. Anxiety, however, is no one's fault. It's not your spouse's fault. It's not your parents' fault. It's not society's fault. It's not your fault. No one is to blame.

You may think you lack willpower because you feel so helpless and terrified. Perhaps you think you should be able to overcome anxiety on your own and not let this thing get the best of you. Well, this isn't true. To have to live with anxiety and simply get through each day has taken great willpower and courage. Many times you felt hopeless and out of control, yet you found the strength to go on.

Men, in particular, often fear being judged as weak, childish, or inferior when suffering from anxiety. Because of chauvinistic attitudes that men are always supposed to be tough and strong, many males think that seeking help implies weakness—a fault that "should" be overcome by personal strength, discipline, and fortitude. For both men and women, seeking help for anxiety does not imply a lack of personal fiber or moral character. To the contrary, it takes great courage to admit you're anxious and go for help.

THE FEAR OF INTIMACY

We all need to love and be loved, yet anxiety about relationships is pervasive. If we have been hurt by painful childhood experiences or been rejected in our adult love relationships, we may be afraid to risk again and be limited by a fear of intimacy.

When a love relationship feels unsafe, we may retreat into our protective shells. Though we long to be appreciated, nurtured, and loved, guarding our affection too closely creates a vicious cycle. The more we fear being open and vulnerable, the more loneliness and frustration persist. The fear of getting hurt blocks our love and keeps us from a secure and lasting intimacy. Which of the following common expressions of the fear of intimacy apply to you?

- "When I get intimately involved, my common sense flies out the window."
- "I worry that my partner will get tired of me."
- "Relationships seem to bring out the worst in me."
- "I'm afraid my career would suffer if I made a commitment to settle down."
- "As soon as it starts to get serious, my doubts appear."
- "Everyone I'm attracted to is either married, in love with someone else, or somehow unavailable."
- "I'm giving too much and getting too little in return."
- "I've been on my own for so long, I couldn't live with someone else."
- "I'm afraid of falling into the same kind of unhappy marriage my parents had."
- "After what I went through with my ex, I'll never be able to trust anyone."
- "I worry that there's something missing in our relationship."

Anxiety impairs the ability to care and be cared for, to love and feel lovable. The anxious person may be so self-absorbed in worries, fears, and emotional pain that loved ones feel neglected or rejected. Anxious people often fail to express their feelings because of the fear of rejection and embarrassment. They rarely respond to annoying matters in their relationships until some minor event becomes the "last straw." Some people think they are anxious because of difficult relationships, but perhaps they have difficult relationships because they are anxious.

Unrecognized anxiety can eat away at relationships and block success. Overprotective loved ones worry about the anxious person's reactions to things. Family members don't know how to deal with the endless worrying and incessant fears. Success implies changes in responsibility, lifestyle, and work, but for anxious people change is frightening. They are reluctant to surrender the safety of the routine and the familiar. The instinct to resist change, to avoid risk-taking and the unfamiliar, overrides the desire to succeed. If anxiety goes untreated, fear and suffering seep into the most intimate aspects of the personality, impairing one's relationship with self, family, friends, coworkers, God, and life.

4

A Worried Mind

*We are, perhaps, uniquely among the earth's
creatures, the worrying animal. We worry
away our lives, fearing the future, discontent
with the present, unable to take in the idea of
dying, unable to sit still.*
                                                    —LEWIS THOMAS, M.D.

Worry is the most common form that anxiety takes. Fearful,
troublesome thoughts can become relentless. Dr. Daniel Goleman suggests, "Chronic worry has all the attributes of a low-
grade emotional high-jacking." The habit of worry becomes
so ingrained that the anxious person can always find something to worry about—uncertainty about finances, social
embarrassment, a failure at work, a fear of illness, rejection in
love, or family problems. Some common worries are:

- "I don't dare do that."
- "I'm too embarrassed."
- "Crowds make me feel uncomfortable."
- "I'm terrified of heights."
- "I can't help feeling frightened."
- "I'm scared of rejection."

- "You can't be too careful."
- "What if. . . ."
- "I could die."
- "A panic attack could happen again."

The worried mind endlessly warns of life's possible perils. Instead of coming up with creative solutions to potential problems, anxious thoughts keep the person stuck in an inflexible, relentless rut.

Some anxious people overcompensate by trying to be happy and positive all the time. This is unnatural and usually counterproductive. Don't be seduced by a "don't worry, be happy" attitude. The power of positive thinking often crashes and burns in the face of anxiety. The advice so often given (e.g., "You have nothing to worry about," "Stop worrying") further reinforces feelings of inadequacy and embarrassment. Overly positive, confidence-preaching people can make anxious people feel even worse. The more they fail to follow the "don't worry, be happy" advice, the more shame and low self-esteem they feel.

Some people use worry as a sign that they are truly caring, loving people. The logic is that if you love someone, you have to worry about them. The more you worry, the more you feel like a good spouse, parent, or friend. It doesn't matter that the worry accomplishes nothing and can become a burden to those worried about.

A valuable distinction needs to be made between effective concern and useless worry. On your worry list may be many causes for genuine concern. If you eat a high-fat diet, smoke cigarettes, and don't exercise, you are at greater risk for a heart attack: valid reasons for concern, no question. The difference between concern and worry lies in your ability to do something about the potential disasters that may lie ahead. Concern leads to action. If you're concerned about your health, make changes in your diet, begin a regular routine of moderate exercise, and stop smoking. Concern is a natural expression of your ability to control your own destiny.

Worry is very different. When you worry, your power to do something about potential problems never really enters into the picture. The opposite is the case—worry arises from feelings of powerlessness. When you worry, you may wonder about all the difficulties your family will face if you lose your job. Or you imagine the crushing pain of a heart attack. Or you envision a panic in your household when you can't afford to buy groceries. In all of these mental pictures is you—in the midst of calamity—incapable of acting.

Fundamental to all worry is a pervasive fear that you have no control over your future. Worry is a self-inflicted punishment for that fear. Few people like to look fear in the eye, especially fear of their own helplessness. No one is proud of trying to escape from fear. Bring on old reliable worry! It disguises the fear and punishes you for refusing to confront it honestly and appropriately.

To reduce worry you have to confront your fear of having no control over your life in difficult circumstances. The key is to transform worry from a signal to do nothing into a signal to do something positive. There are some aspects of life over which you have little or no control, so why waste your energy on useless worry? It's wiser to treat these uncertainties like the weather. Accept them and go on to more positive things.

INSOMNIA

Insomnia is a gross feeder. It will nourish itself on any kind of thinking, including thinking about not thinking.

—CLIFTON FADIMAN

Most people who worry also have insomnia because anxiety interrupts sleep and causes nightmares. Difficulty falling asleep or staying asleep, also called intermittent awakening, is often symptomatic of anxiety. Early morning waking (when one awakes at three or four in the morning and is unable to get back to sleep) is more often a symptom of depression. About a third of people with insomnia have an underlying anxiety disorder or a clinical depression.

Mostly, insomnia is transient, typically occurring before a public performance, a major business meeting, or the beginning of a new job. If someone has suffered a significant loss, such as a divorce or the death of a loved one, insomnia can persist for several weeks. Chronic insomnia can be a serious problem for months and even years. Night after night you lie awake tossing and turning, frustrated, muscles tight, mind racing; perhaps you finally get an hour or two of fitful, troubled rest, but upon awakening you feel exhausted. People with chronic insomnia report feelings of apprehension, anxious thoughts, and worry about not sleeping. Sleep loss can lead to irritability, poor concentration, and impaired memory.

Over seventy million Americans have difficulty sleeping; we are becoming a society of sleep-deprived zombies. According to William Dement, M.D., Chairman of the Sleep Disorder Clinic at the Stanford University School of Medicine, "A substantial number of Americans, perhaps the majority, are functionally handicapped by sleep deprivation on any given day." The incidence of insomnia among adults is 30 to 40 percent; one of every five patients seeing a doctor complains of a sleep disorder. A thorough medical examination is always necessary to check for any organic illness, including apnea or narcolepsy. Prescription drugs, such as asthma medications, steroids, and some antidepressants, and over-the-counter products, such as appetite suppressants, nasal decongestants, and nicotine, can cause insomnia. Other causes of insomnia, such as noise, caffeine, alcohol, and cigarettes should also be ruled out. Anxiety produces a viscious circle, where we lie awake worrying about sleep and fearing insomnia.

Natural self-healing techniques of sleep-promoting behavior should always be practiced before considering any pharmaceutical drugs or herbal sleep aids (see Part 3). Unfortunately, insomnia caused by anxiety is often inappropriately treated with sleeping pills. Synthetic drugs to induce sleep often create more problems than they solve. With long-term use they can be addictive and are associated with numerous side effects, including memory loss and morning hangover. People who take benzodiazepine sleeping pills for more than two weeks and then stop suffer frequently from rebound insomnia and vivid nightmares. One-fourth of all cases of insomnia are complicated by withdrawal reactions from synthetic sleeping pills. The advantages of herbal sleep remedies will be explored in Part 2.

5

The Primary Types of Anxiety Disorder

When you think of anxiety, think of Woody Allen; when you think of panic, think of the Last Judgment.
— BARBARA GRIZZUTI HARRISON

Three of every four people with an anxiety disorder are not correctly diagnosed and treated. Yet early recognition and treatment can prevent much unnecessary suffering and help people to recover fully. Following are the primary types of anxiety disorder.

Panic (Anxiety) Attack: A sudden experience of apprehension or terror, often associated with a fear of going crazy, losing control, or impending doom. Heart palpitations, shortness of breath, choking, smothering sensations, chest pain, or light-headedness are other frequent symptoms. The attacks reach their peak in about ten minutes but leave the person scared and emotionally exhausted.

Generalized Anxiety Disorder (GAD): Persistent anxiety and worry for at least six months, characterized by restlessness, irritability, muscle tension, fatigue, sleep disturbance, or difficulty concentrating. The anxiety and worry cause distress or impairment in school, work, and social activities. The person almost constantly worries about something and expects the worst to happen.

Phobia: Persistent, unreasonable fear that is triggered by the presence or anticipation of a specific object or situation. The phobic stimulus is avoided or endured with dread. Phobia has three major subcategories:

- *Simple or Specific Phobias:* These phobias are characterized by intense, unfounded, and enduring fear of a specific object or activity. For instance, some people suffer from an elevator phobia, although the odds of being killed in an elevator are one in seventeen million. Other common phobias are fear of flying, heights, dogs, snakes, mice, spiders, seeing blood, or receiving an injection. People with simple or specific phobias usually develop anticipatory anxiety at the prospect of facing whatever object or situation they fear and will do anything to avoid it.
- *Social Phobia:* A marked fear of public humiliation or embarrassment in social or performance situations like public speaking or taking a test. Sufferers will do anything they can to avoid the situations they fear.
- *Agoraphobia:* An abnormal fear of open or public places, such as a fear of being in crowds, riding in cars, or entering an elevator, situations or places from which it might be difficult or embarrassing to escape. Agoraphobics fear that help may be unavailable if a panic attack occurs and so avoid these circumstances.

Obsessive-Compulsive Disorder (OCD): Recurrent obsessions—such as intrusive, persistent thoughts, images, or impulses—or compulsions—such as repetitive behaviors (like ritualized hand-washing, cleaning, or list-making), checking (repeated checking of door locks and appliances, making mistakes, or causing possible damage), or ordering (extreme concern for exactness, symmetry, or repetitive counting)—that cause marked anxiety and consume more than an hour a day. OCD is as common an illness as asthma or diabetes, affecting about six million people annually.

Post-Traumatic Stress Disorder (PTSD): The experience or witnessing of events causing profound emotional trauma, such as torture, rape, or threat of death, followed by recurrent flashbacks of the traumatic event. It can also involve nightmares, eating disorders, terror, fatigue, forgetfulness, withdrawal, and hypervigilance.

Hypochondriasis: Unwarranted fear of having a serious disease. The person persists in misinterpreting or exaggerating bodily symptoms despite appropriate medical evaluation and reassurance. This obsession with illness may be a type of OCD.

Dysmorphophobia: Persistent fears of being ugly; complaints centering on fears that the face, body, limbs, or sex organs are misshapen. Sufferers worry that others comment adversely about their appearance, even after plastic surgery to correct the imagined stigma. Some researchers consider the fixation on perceived flaws in appearance to also be a variation of OCD.

Please remember that while you may have an anxiety disorder, *you* are not disordered. Once recognized and accepted, an anxiety disorder is highly treatable. Diagnosis is part of a process to diminish your symptoms, not yourself.

PANIC ATTACK

According to the American Psychiatric Association,[1] a panic attack is a discrete period of intense fear in which at least four of the following symptoms develop abruptly and reach a peak within ten minutes:

- Palpitations, accelerated heart rate
- Sweating
- Trembling or shaking
- Sensations of shortness of breath or smothering
- Feeling of choking
- Chest pain or discomfort
- Nausea or abdominal distress
- Feeling dizzy, unsteady, light-headed, or faint
- Feelings of unreality or being detached from oneself
- Fear of losing control or going crazy
- Fear of dying
- Numbness or tingling sensations
- Chills or hot flashes

Fear begets fear. Anticipatory anxiety develops from worrying about the occurrence of another panic attack. As a result, a third of those with a panic disorder develop agoraphobia.

HYPERVENTILATION

Anxiety can leave you breathless. The symptoms of hyperventilation, which literally means overbreathing, are commonly experienced by people with anxiety and yet frequently go unrecognized by either the doctor or the sufferer. Yet hyperventilation accounts for over 10 percent of visits to hospital emergency rooms.

Although breathing is the most fundamental function of being alive, many people breathe improperly. Rapid, shallow breathing leads to exhaling too much carbon dioxide, which can produce many frightening sensations including light-headedness, dizziness, shortness of breath, perspiration, numbness and tingling, and chest pain.

An increase in the rapidity and tightness of breathing may be so slight as to go unobserved. A respiratory rate greater than fifteen breaths per minute generally indicates hyperventilation, especially if accompanied by frequent sighing and yawning. Medical causes of hyperventilation, such as asthma, bronchitis, and heart disease, should always be ruled out. Worry, stress, and poor posture are by far the most common precipitants. Hyperventilation can trigger a panic attack and tends to run in families.

Relaxation and breath retraining are skills essential to treating hyperventilation and healing anxiety (see chapter 24). Learning to breathe abdominally with an erect posture is a powerful tool for reducing stress and anxiety instantly. Regular physical activity also leads to deeper breathing and expelling the proper amount of carbon dioxide. In an emergency, breathe into a paper lunch bag, which you hold with both hands over your nose and mouth. Recycling the same air allows more exhaled carbon dioxide to be inhaled. After ten or more slow, natural breaths, you will be able to breathe normally again.

ANXIETY CAN FEEL LIFE-THREATENING

Anxiety signals a threat to one's well-being. Feeling out of control, the anxious person starts to anticipate the worst possible consequences: "I can't breathe" or "I'm having a stroke." About 10 percent of visits to the emergency room for a possible heart attack are actually due to the symptoms of a panic attack—shortness of breath, chest pain, rapid heartbeat, dizziness, sweating, and fear of impending doom. People with obsessive-compulsive disorder are hyperaware of potential threats to health and well-being. While the symptoms of anxiety are distressing, they do not indicate a grave illness. Even without treatment, the symptoms will eventually diminish. No one has ever died of an anxiety attack. The fear will pass; you will survive.

Of course, if you fear you are having a heart attack, don't assume that it's "only anxiety." It is best to go to a hospital emergency room for a diagnosis. If, after a complete medical evaluation, you are found to be physically healthy, accept the reassurance. Anxiety can feel life-threatening, but you will survive and get better. The healing process has a beginning, a middle, and an end.

6

What Causes Anxiety?

In view of the intimate connection between things physical and mental, we may look forward to the day when paths of knowledge will be opened up leading from organic biology and chemistry to the field of neurotic phenomena.

—SIGMUND FREUD

Recent scientific research suggests that anxiety is the result of a biochemical imbalance in the brain's alarm center—the amygdala—and a psychological imbalance in thinking. The combination of a biochemically overreactive amygdala and fearful, worrisome thinking causes an exaggerated and persistent stress response. As to which comes first, this is a little like the chicken-or-the-egg question. The answer is both, in a circular pattern of causation. This is the mind-body principle: every change in the mind (anxiety) produces a corresponding change in the body (alarm) and vice versa.

While treatment of a biochemical imbalance solely with drugs is often assumed to be successful, research has shown that cognitive psychotherapy (correcting distorted thinking) can also cause an immediate and lasting correction in brain chemistry. This has been illustrated by brain imagery studies performed at major medical centers.

Anxiety can be the result of a number of factors—genetic predisposition, a painful childhood, major stress or trauma, medical illness, alcohol or drug abuse—and can also occur for no obvious or apparent reason.

THE AMYGDALA— THE BRAIN'S ALARM CENTER

Located in the emotional center of the brain, the amygdala signals trouble instantaneously, like a neural tripwire. It telegraphs a message of crisis before the cortex, the thinking area of your brain, is able to check whether or not the threat is real. The amygdala alarm center has proven to be life-saving throughout the primeval dangers of humanity's evolution, but it can also produce false alarms—unnecessary fear, anxiety, and worry. Experiences that frighten us the most produce high arousal in the amygdala, imprinting indelible emotional memories. Anything remotely similar to a past trauma can trigger an emergency response in the amygdala. An adjacent area, the caudate nucleus, has been shown to be overactive in obsessive-compulsive disorder.

A hypersensitive amygdala can lead to worry run amok. Overstimulation of the amygdala through chronic repetitive stress or an acute major trauma can cause it to remain excessively aroused and overreactive. As a result, the amygdala can trigger a five-alarm fire in response to a little bit of smoke or no threat at all. The lower alarm threshold can trigger a panic reaction to any arousal, whether physical (as from exercising) or emotional (hearing news of an accident involving a loved one). Even awakening to an alarm clock can be so jarring that it triggers anxiety.

NEUROTRANSMITTERS—
THE MESSENGERS
OF THE BRAIN

The human brain is the most complex, intricate communication center known to us, transmitting billions of messages each second without our thinking about it. The biochemical messengers of this communication are known as *neurotransmitters*. (*Neuro* refers to the brain and *transmitter* to sending and receiving information.)

When neurotransmitters are at appropriate levels, the brain functions harmoniously and the overall mood is one of well-being, confidence, and ease. Serotonin is an especially important neurotransmitter that can act as the brain's own tranquilizer and antidepressant. Low serotonin levels have been implicated in anxiety, worry, panic, premenstrual syndrome (PMS), social phobia, depression, and impulsive disorders (such as violence, stealing, shopping, gambling, and overeating). Anxiety disorders may reflect serotonin deficits in the amygdala. The reason selective serotonin reuptake inhibitors (SSRIs) and the herb Saint-John's-wort (see chapter 13) are effective in treating anxiety is that they correct serotonin imbalances in the amygdala.

There is also significant evidence associating anxiety (panic) attacks with another neurotransmitter, norepinephrine, which is released by the brain in emergencies. Impaired balance of norepinephrine and serotonin can cause a panic attack. Many high-strung, fearful people have low levels of another neurotransmitter, gamma-aminobutyric acid (GABA). The herbs valerian and kava can enhance the action of GABA, thereby reducing anxiety and nervous tension.

ANXIETY CAN BE
HEREDITARY AND CONTAGIOUS

A predisposition to anxiety can be hereditary. Serotonin and other brain chemicals are affected by our genes, as well as by our attitudes, experiences, and spirit. The risk of panic attacks is about eight times higher among close relatives than in the general population. Life is full of stressful events, many of which cannot and should not be avoided, which can trigger anxiety in those who are susceptible. As with many illnesses, such as heart disease and diabetes, anxiety disorders can run in the family. Children who receive the affected gene are more vulnerable to anxiety than others.

What makes people susceptible to a hypersensitive amygdala is complex, but genetics can play a role. Research has identified a gene on chromosome 17 that contributes to neuroticism and a gene on chromosome 22 appears to be linked to obsessive-compulsive disorder. About 40 percent of people with agoraphobia have a relative with an anxiety disorder. Also, if one of a pair of identical twins suffers from panic disorder, there is a 40 percent chance the other suffers as well.

Having the genes for an anxiety disorder does not mean that heredity is destiny. Environmental factors and a resilient spirit are just as important. Many people with a genetic predisposition do not develop an anxiety disorder, while others without a family history do so. An interplay of biological, behavioral, and psychosocial factors determines whether or not anxiety becomes a problem. Of course, as Vladimir Nabokov writes, "Neither in environment nor in heredity can I find the exact instrument that fashioned me."

Physical, emotional, and sexual abuse are known precipitants of anxiety. If guilt, shame, fear, and hostility were regularly used by parents to control a child's behavior, that child is more likely to grow up fearful and lacking in confidence.

Family-of-origin difficulties can be a cause of unconscious conflict and chronic anxiety.

Increased irritability is a hallmark of anxiety. The smallest incidents, such as a misplaced phone message or spilled milk on the kitchen floor, can lead to a tirade or temper outburst. Perhaps as a result of this emotional instability and unpredictability, an anxious person who is married has a much greater likelihood of having an anxious spouse. Is it *assortive mating* (the tendency to pair off with someone who has the same problem) or is it that the anxiety of an anxious spouse can be "contagious"? In either case, it seems that misery does love company.

Studies indicate that anxious people are very susceptible to taking on the negative emotions of those around them. Whenever you feel anxious, check to see if you are in the presence of a complainer. When you can't move away or find a more positive conversational focus, you might put on an imaginary emotional raincoat, or create a picture of protecting yourself from the energy-depleting rain of stressful words. In this way you are likely to be less vulnerable to contagious negativity. The other person's mood has little or nothing to do with you. When you allow hurtful or irritating words to get inside you and fester, you are torturing yourself needlessly.

CHILDHOOD ANXIETY AND ATTENTION DEFICIT DISORDER

About one in five infants is born with a timid temperament. These infants are fearful and overly sensitive, which makes them vulnerable to developing persistent separation anxiety—a fear of being separated from parents or being away from home. They cry, beg, and cling whenever left alone. In grade school, timid children talk less, are shy in social situations, and are terrified of choking up for a class speech or school performance. Research indicates that shyness, fear of strangers, social introversion, and excessive fear of embarrassment are personality traits that can be inherited.

Attention deficit disorder (ADD)—being easily distracted and having difficulty paying attention—and attention deficit hyperactivity disorder (ADHD)—also being fidgety, aggressive, and "bouncing off the walls"—may overlap with anxiety and depression. There are probably multiple causes of these symptom complexes—genetic, neurological, temperamental, nutritional, and social. ADD/ADHD is the most common psychiatric diagnosis in childhood. About 50 percent of these children continue to have attention and behavioral problems in adolescence (such as juvenile delinquency, drug abuse, and school difficulties), and 25 percent continue to have persistent symptoms into adulthood.

Specialized education, behavioral strategies, dietary changes, and synthetic drugs can be of benefit. Herbal remedies can be helpful in the treatment of ADD/ADHD when used with other supportive measures (see chapter 14). Certainly more natural medicines should be considered before automatically dosing a child or adolescent with Ritalin (methylphenidate), an addictive drug that can have significant side effects and unknown long-term consequences.

7

The Diagnosis
of Anxiety

*I observe the physician with the same dili-
gence as he the disease.*

—JOHN DONNE

About 70 percent of people with anxiety have consulted
more than ten physicians (e.g., internists, cardiologists, gas-
troenterologists, emergency room doctors) before the cause
of their racing heart, difficult breathing, fainting, trembling,
or aching stomach is correctly diagnosed. Many general
practitioners and nonpsychiatric specialists are too busy or
too focused on their specialty to diagnose anxiety accurately.
Anxiety is best diagnosed by a psychiatrist, psychologist, or
other mental health specialist.

Diagnosing anxiety, from the patient's point of view, is an
uncomplicated, straightforward procedure. There will probably be forms to complete concerning your medical and personal history. Be sure to report to the doctor all possible
symptoms of anxiety, and answer all the doctor's questions as
frankly as possible. Because anxiety tends to run in families,
you will be asked about your family medical history.

You should discuss all of the medications and recreational drugs you have taken recently. Prescription drugs such as certain antidepressants—Prozac (fluoxetine), Wellbutrin (bupropion), and Norpramin (desipramine)—steroids, theophylline (an asthma medication), thyroid pills, over-the-counter medications such as diet pills and decongestants, and illicit drugs such as amphetamines, cocaine, and narcotics can cause or worsen anxiety. Also, coffee (excess caffeine), cigarette smoking, and MSG (monosodium glutamate) can trigger anxiety.

Many drugs, both pharmaceuticals and abused substances, can produce anxiety not only while being taken but also when suddenly withdrawn. Benzodiazepines, which are frequently prescribed for anxiety relief and sleep, can be addictive and cause rebound anxiety and insomnia when discontinued. As will be detailed in Part 2, natural tranquilizers such as kava and valerian can be safely used for a longer period and are not addictive. When discontinued, these natural substances do not cause withdrawal symptoms.

It is important to receive a medical checkup to rule out physical illnesses that may cause anxiety. For example, people with mitral valve prolapse, a usually benign abnormality of the heart valve, are prone to suffer panic attacks. Other medical conditions that can cause anxiety are coronary heart disease, emphysema, hyperventilation, hyperthyroidism, and anemia. Most of these conditions can be diagnosed by laboratory tests and a physical examination.

Some people may have an anxiety disorder without necessarily *feeling* unusual amounts of fear or apprehension. Their major symptoms can be exclusively physical—sweating, upset stomach, dizziness, light-headedness, numbness or tingling of the hands or feet, diarrhea, hyperventilation, flushing, twitching, exhaustion, a lump in the throat, or insomnia.

Anxiety can cause a wide variety of symptoms affecting every part of the body, sometimes making it very difficult to diagnose. People often consult many different specialists but after many expensive laboratory tests and checkups still go undiagnosed, in part because anxiety is a great impostor. It can be disguised and look like many other illnesses. Anxiety can be blocked or denied on the emotional level and present only as physical distress. The organ that is the focus of bodily complaint is usually one particularly subject to physiological expressions of anxiety; for example, the heart or bowel.

Anxiety may also be masked by obsessive-compulsive behavior, such as repeated hand-washing and checking for uncleanliness. Compulsive rituals may become so severe that they interfere with social functioning, intimate relationships, and work adjustment and yet not be realistically associated with anxiety and distress. Obsessions about food, dieting, and exercise may be used to avoid feeling anxious about body image. Some people refuse to relax or avoid being alone in order to keep their suppressed fears from surfacing. Obsessive-compulsive personality disorder involves a chronic preoccupation with precision, orderliness, perfectionism, and control. In moderation these traits are not only normal but perhaps desirable for achievement and success. When these qualities become inflexible and pervasive, they can give rise to a disorder. Obsessive-compulsive disorder is a specific illness characterized by intrusive recurrent obsessions and distressing compulsive rituals.

ANXIETY, ALCOHOLISM, AND ADDICTIONS

There are probably people who are considered alcoholic who only drink to control their anxiety disease. When this

*is treated successfully, their strong urge to drink lessens.
The alcoholism is really only secondary to the anxiety disease, a complication of it.*
                              —DAVID V. SHEEHAN, M.D.

Left untreated, anxiety can be a pervasive source of misery emotionally, mentally, and physically. Some people seek
relief in alcohol or drugs. Alcohol is the most commonly self-
prescribed sedative for anxiety. It is readily available and
socially acceptable. Unfortunately, alcohol only worsens the
condition when it is taken in the quantities some consume to
obtain mental and emotional oblivion. Anxiety can also be
caused by alcohol withdrawal.

Drugs of all kinds—legal, illegal, over-the-counter, or
prescription—are sometimes inappropriately used by anxious people in an attempt to numb themselves. Opiate
painkillers, tranquilizers, cocaine, and amphetamines are not
only ineffective but often make the anxiety worse.

Many people when they are under pressure engage in
oral activities like overeating, drinking, smoking, nail-biting,
and pencil chewing as "oral tranquilizers." Other common
nervous habits are hair pulling, eye blinking, throat clearing,
coughing, stuttering, and teeth grinding (bruxism). Anxiety
can also lead to other habitual, often addictive behavior, such
as compulsive shopping, stealing, gambling, and sex.

Fearful negative thoughts can also become a bad habit.
Any disturbing thought can become repetitive and spiral out
of control even though you may realize that worrying does
not help.

ANXIETY AND DEPRESSION

Pain is inevitable. Suffering is optional.
> —M. KATHLEEN CASEY

Anxiety can become progressively disabling at work and in personal relationships. Anxious people have frequent feelings of guilt and worthlessness about not being able to cope successfully with situations that other people have no difficulty with and about being dependent on family and friends, thereby restricting their lives. The longer anxiety persists without effective treatment, the more likely it is that those who suffer will become depressed. As anxiety becomes progressively more disabling, it can significantly hamper the ability to live a full and enjoyable life.

Anxiety and depression frequently occur in tandem. Irritability, difficulty concentrating, indecision, guilt, fatigue, sleep and eating disturbances, and chronic aches and pains are symptoms common to both disorders. In particular, agoraphobia and depression are closely linked. Almost half of the people who suffer repeated panic attacks develop a major case of depression. Low levels of serotonin have been implicated in both anxiety disorders and depression. Many studies have found that selective serotonin reuptake inhibitors (SSRIs), such as Prozac (fluoxetine), Paxil (paroxetine), and Anafranil (clomipramine), are useful in treating both anxiety and depression. The natural antidepressant herb Saint-John's-wort can be effective not only for depression but also for anxiety.

Clinical depression is a specific illness that requires intervention. According to the National Institute of Mental Health, symptoms of clinical depression can include:

- Chronically sad or "empty" mood
- Lack of interest or pleasure in ordinary activities, including sex

- Decreased energy, fatigue; being "slowed down"
- Sleep disturbances (insomnia, early morning waking, or oversleeping)
- Eating disturbances (loss of appetite and weight, or weight gain)
- Difficulty concentrating, remembering, or making decisions
- Feelings of guilt, worthlessness, and helplessness
- Thoughts of death or suicide; suicide attempts
- Irritability, lack of cooperation
- Excessive crying
- Chronic aches and pains that don't respond to treatment
- Decreased productivity, lack of cooperation
- Safety problems, accidents
- Alcohol or drug abuse

A thorough diagnosis is needed if four or more of these symptoms persist for more than two weeks or are interfering with work or family life. Consult a qualified mental health professional for a professional diagnosis. Clinical depression is different from the pain that immediately follows a loss and from the down cycle in life's ordinary ups and downs. Nor does clinical depression reflect the popular use of the word *depressed*, which usually means feeling disappointed or temporarily dejected. There are three major forms of clinical depression:

- *Major depression:* Like pneumonia, major depression has a beginning, a middle, and an end. Untreated, the average episode of major depression lasts six months, and it can return periodically for an average of five to six episodes in a lifetime.
- *Dysthymia (chronic depression):* If a depression is experienced most of the day, more days than not, for more than two years, it's known as dysthymia. Dysthymia lasts more than five years on average if it goes untreated.

- *Manic-depression (bipolar illness):* Here the lows of depression can alternate with *mania*—extreme elation, unreasonably grandiose thoughts, sleeplessness, reckless hyperactivity, and inappropriate, sometimes destructive actions. Manic episodes return more or less regularly unless they are treated.

People who suffer from clinical depression have significant amounts of physical, psychological, and occupational disability. Depressive symptoms may also occur under specific circumstances, such as seasonal affective disorder (SAD), premenstrual syndrome (PMS), postpartum blues or depression, and bereavement (melancholia), as a consequence of drug and alcohol abuse, and as a result of medical conditions like low thyroid disease. A practical guide to consult is a book I coauthored with Peter McWilliams, *How to Heal Depression* (Prelude Press, 1994).

8

Anxiety Is an Exaggerated Stress Response

Any time you get upset it tears down your nervous system.

—MAE WEST

In engineering, the word *stress* refers to a force sufficient to distort or deform when applied to a system. The modern usage of *stress* refers to the wear and tear of fast-paced living. Hans Selye, Ph.D., a Canadian endocrinologist, discovered the common set of physiological changes that occur whenever a person experiences difficulties or undue pressures. He called these changes, technically, the *general adaptation syndrome*, or more simply, *the stress response*. Dr. Selye defined *stress* as the nonspecific response of the body to any demand made upon it, whether physical, mental, or emotional.

In his groundbreaking research, Dr. Selye demonstrated that the body responds with the same characteristic set of changes to a loud noise, a sudden temperature drop, a viral infection, intense pleasure, worry, or difficulties at work. Not just a response of one organ or one part of the body, the stress response involves a predictable set of physical consequences. Some of the bodily changes that accompany stress include muscular tension, increased heart rate, accelerated breathing, mild to profuse sweating, and cold hands or feet. When the stress response becomes exaggerated (i.e., intense and prolonged), it can cause anxiety.

The stress response in itself is neither good nor bad. In fact, making value judgments about inborn biological responses is usually a mistake. Whatever nature has built into the body almost always has a useful function. The mild excitation caused by the stress response to life's challenges allows you to make a successful adaptation. A small amount of stress, over a limited period of time, is a natural part of change and growth. This sense of mild excitation can enhance creativity and stimulate peak performance. Dr. Selye called this healthy level of stress *eustress.* You could not defend against a bacterial invasion, work hard, experience great joy and excitement, or delight in sexual pleasure and orgasm without the stress response. Clearly this response is fundamental to your survival and "thrival," your enjoyment of living. But research has shown that when the stress response is intense and prolonged, what Selye called *distress,* it can erode the foundations of your health.

It is important to distinguish between debilitating stress and a healthy state of high arousal. Actors often get butterflies before going on stage. Athletes get psyched up before a competition. Effective speakers may feel excitement before giving an important speech. This high-arousal state is physically akin to the anxiety that causes so much distress in everyday life, but there is an important distinction. A high-arousal state energizes and mobilizes you for a peak effort, but everyday stress, anxiety, and worry dissipate energy in useless fretting and can wear down your nervous system. Of course, striving for no stress is not the answer; you soon become bored, and boredom in itself can cause anxiety. Either extreme, being overstimulated or understimulated, can precipitate anxiety.

In the past, physical hardships such as freezing weather, inadequate nutrition, and frequent illness caused excessive stress and resulted in physical deterioration. These physical hardships are no longer prevalent in postindustrial societies, but new causes of distress—the by-products of modern civilization—have become commonplace. These include physical factors, such as noise, foul air, and hurry to meet rushed schedules, and emotional ones, including financial worries, frustrations at work, and marital strife. Equally important are spiritual problems, such as inner emptiness and lack of fulfillment. With the increase in material well-being that has accompanied the growth of modern civilization, major infectious diseases, such as smallpox and diphtheria, have all but disappeared. The ravages of prolonged stress, however, have never been greater.

What are the symptoms of excessive stress? One common symptom is feeling worn out, emotionally exhausted, at the end of the day. Another is difficulty falling asleep or intermittently awaking throughout the night. Others include:

- Tension headaches
- Chronic fatigue
- Feeling wound up
- Feeling down in the dumps
- Worrying
- Pouches or dark circles under the eyes
- Inability to concentrate
- Irritability
- Frequent indigestion
- Frequent constipation or loose stools

- Frequent colds or flu infections
- Frequent angry outbursts
- Excessive drinking, smoking, or eating

THE STRESS SCALE

Indicate how strongly you agree with each of the following statements on a scale from 0 to 3:

> 0 = never
> 1 = sometimes
> 2 = often
> 3 = always

- I have trouble relaxing.
- I get frustrated when people are incompetent.
- I feel tense and rushed.
- I worry about work and other problems.
- I have difficulty falling asleep.
- I feel grief or loss.
- I am exhausted by daily demands at work and home.
- I feel stuck in a rat race.
- No matter how hard I try, I never feel caught up.
- I feel burdened by financial obligations.
- I am under strain at work.
- I feel lonely and unloved.
- I am embarrassed to ask for assistance.
- I feel overwhelmed by my responsibilities.
- I can't stand criticism.
- I'm afraid I'll lose my job or livelihood.
- People let me down.
- No matter what I achieve, I feel dissatisfied.
- I stew in my anger rather than express it.
- I feel apprehensive about the future.

- My stress is caused by forces beyond my control.
- I feel pressured by my commitments.
- I have difficulty delegating.
- I feel like running away.
- My mind is churning and busy.

Scoring
57 to 75 = high stress; life feels like one crisis after another
38 to 56 = moderate stress; you often feel trapped and out of control
19 to 37 = mild stress; you have some apprehension and struggle
0 to 18 = you are resilient and feel in charge of your life

Regardless of what causes stress, once the reaction gets triggered, your body goes through a response, general adaptation syndrome, that unfolds in three stages.

THE ALARM REACTION: "FIGHT OR FLIGHT"

The first stage of the stress response alarm, also called "fight or flight," is the body's natural reaction to a perceived threat or a real impending danger. If while crossing the street you have to dodge an unexpected automobile, the alarm response provides the instantaneous burst of energy you need to survive.

When a person meets a stressful situation, the brain's alarm center, the amygdala, signals the pituitary, the master gland of the body. The pituitary then sends hormonal messages to the adrenal glands, sitting atop the kidneys. Immediately the adrenals secrete adrenaline and noradrenaline for a massive mobilization of energy, potentially to fight for your life or flee danger. Excess adrenaline can tear the artery walls, damaging them and leaving places for the blood fats to lodge. Excess adrenaline can also overcontract and rupture heart muscle fibers, weakening the heart and making it vulnerable to an electrical short circuit.

The alarm reaction in mild and occasionally intense forms can add joie de vivre or frustration, depending on how you view the situation. Watching a thrilling football game and fighting rush hour traffic may produce the same intensity of stress response, but the football game results in excitement while the traffic jam can cause irritation. Stress becomes negative and debilitating when you perceive change and pressure as a burden and rising demands as a threat, when you perceive yourself as the victim of circumstances, increasingly powerless over the events of your life.

RESISTANCE — THE BODY'S DEFENSE AGAINST STRESS

If the external battle remains or if you continue to trigger stress through worry and frustration, you enter the stage of resistance. This second stage of the stress response is a double-edged sword. It helps you to defend against and resist illness and prolonged hardship. But repeated or prolonged negative stress may lead to an exhaustion of mental and physical energies and increase susceptibility to disease.

During the resistance stage, the pituitary gland secretes hormones that mobilize your whole body for a long-term battle:

- One of these hormones, vasopressin, raises your blood pressure by causing arteries to constrict.

- Another, thyrotropic hormone, stimulates your thyroid gland to increase production of the hormone thyroxine, accelerating your metabolism.
- A third pituitary hormone, called adrenocorticotrophic hormone (ACTH), further activates your adrenal glands to produce cortisol, which, among other effects, raises your blood sugar level, alters your immune system, and increases blood platelets (blood-clotting elements), which can adhere to artery walls, narrowing them.

The body draws on available nutrients and reserves of energy to fuel the stage of resistance. When stress is prolonged, the body forms *free radicals*, undesirable chemicals that have long been implicated in degenerative diseases and hastening the aging process. When the body's energy reserves become depleted, the adrenal glands can no longer function efficiently. The result can be a decreased ability to cope with stress and chronic anxiety. The second stage of the stress response, however, need not be damaging. If not prolonged, it will naturally give way to the third stage, exhaustion, during which the body can replenish its biochemical resources.

EMOTIONAL AND PHYSICAL EXHAUSTION

The expenditure of energy and vital bodily resources in the first two stages leads to exhaustion, the third phase of the stress response. This fatigue persists until the body can achieve deep rest and replenish itself. Fatigue is the number one complaint heard in doctors' offices. More than 40 percent of general medical patients complain that they feel too exhausted to perform at their best and enjoy their lives. The signs and symptoms of chronic fatigue are as follows:

- Dullness
- Poor muscle tone
- Pasty, pale complexion
- Lack of spontaneity
- Tendency to be bored or depressed
- Fear, tension, and anxiety
- Decreased cooperativeness
- Less acceptance of constructive criticism
- Irritability, temper outbursts
- Lowered attention span
- Impaired recent memory
- Decreased sex drive
- Insomnia, waking up tired
- Physical complaints, such as headache or back pain
- Decreased interest in personal care
- Addiction to coffee, cigarettes, and stimulants
- Alcohol and drug abuse
- Decreased general health and satisfaction

When the body does not receive sufficient rest to restore its equilibrium, stress can disrupt the innate biological rhythms on which health and productivity depend—waking, dreaming, and sleeping. While awake, the stressed person feels agitated and exhausted. When dreaming, the stressed person has night-mares. While asleep, the stressed person is restless and awakes unrefreshed. In this deenergized but uptight state, problems seem ever more daunting. There's a greater tendency for self-defeating thoughts and behaviors. You may try to appear calm, but feigning tranquillity doesn't relieve the pressure.

Relaxation does not mean depleted energy or dulled senses. By developing your ability to quickly enter a state of profound, revitalizing relaxation—restful alertness—you can distance yourself from life's noise and distractions and promote greater clear-mindedness and awareness (see Part 3).

DIS-EASE AND DIS-ORDER

If this essential core of the person is denied or suppressed, he gets sick sometimes in obvious ways, sometimes in subtle ways, sometimes immediately, sometimes later.
                    —ABRAHAM MASLOW, PH.D.

Medical research has repeatedly demonstrated that stress causes, contributes to, and aggravates anxiety disorders and physical illnesses. A landmark Harvard study[1] showed that people who cope poorly with stress become ill four times more often than those with good coping styles. Chronic distress can lead to the following:

- General muscular tension, with increased headaches and back pain/stiffness
- Suppression of the immune system, with a reduction of the white blood cells critically important to fighting a cold, flu, or even cancer and shrinking of the thymus, spleen, and lymph nodes
- Chronic elevation of blood pressure with slow, steady damage to the heart, kidneys, and entire cardiovascular system
- Increase in abdominal fat
- Increased "bad" low-density lipoproteins (LDL), leading to an increased cholesterol level
- Depletion of calcium from the bones
- Spasms of the gastrointestinal tract, which can lead to irritable bowel or spastic colon
- Excess secretion of stomach acid, which can leave you vulnerable to a peptic ulcer
- Tearing of arterial walls and elevation of clotting elements in the blood, both of which increase plaque formation (clogging) in the arteries
- Increased heart rate and electrical conduction problems,

which can cause cardiac arrhythmias
- Decline in sex hormones
- Killing of brain cells, premature aging of the brain, and interference with neurotransmitter function
- Significant decreases in learning ability, memory, concentration, and even IQ

If you experience distress only occasionally, it will do little permanent damage. But if you experience excessive long-term stress on a daily basis, it will profoundly disturb your health. Chronic stress can contribute to serious illnesses, such as heart disease and cancer. Mortality rises sharply among people with prolonged stress. The emotional consequences of chronic stress are as harmful as the physical ones. They may be even more dangerous because they inhibit your coping ability, which leads to more stress. Prolonged stress keeps your nervous system hyperaroused, resulting in anxiety.

CHRONIC TENSION

There are two primary energy states. The one in which most of us are trapped is called *tense energy*, which is a state of high tension and high energy. The other, which most of us have lost touch with, is called *calm energy*, which is a state of low tension and high energy.

Tense energy is a stress-driven mood characterized by an almost pleasant sense of excitement and power. Your physical energy feels high, even though you may face a high level of stress and strain from long hours of a hectic work schedule. In a tense energy state, you tend to push yourself impatiently toward one objective after another, rarely pausing to rest or reflect. Your efforts are infused with a moderate to severe level of physical tension, which after a while may be imperceptible to you. When tense energy persists, you can suddenly wake up to find yourself on the verge of a panic attack.

Calm energy is a state that few of us experience often enough. Calm energy feels remarkably serene and under control. It replaces tense energy with peaceful, pleasurable body feelings and an alert, optimistic presence of mind. When you are in a calm energy state, your mental and physical reserves are high, and you have the best combination of healthy vitality and increased creative intelligence. Calm energy breeds the confidence, optimism, and stamina necessary for success. In Part 3 I will outline strategies and techniques to cultivate calm energy.

PART 2

HERBS FOR ANXIETY, INSOMNIA, AND STRESS

God who sends the wound sends the medicine.
—CERVANTES

9

The Herbal
Medicine Revolution

*If you are herbally inclined, you might ask
your physicians which pharmaceuticals they
would recommend for your ailment, then
ask whether there is any proof that they are
better than the herbal alternative.*
— JAMES A. DUKE, PH.D.,
THE GREEN PHARMACY

The World Health Organization estimates that 80 percent of the people on earth rely on herbs for their health care needs. Widespread usage of medicinal herbs is no longer limited to third world countries. In many countries, including Germany, France, Italy, Japan, and Australia, herbal products are commonly taken as supplements as well as prescribed in medical practice. In 1996 Americans spent three and one-quarter billion dollars on herbal remedies, still less than the six billion dollars spent by Germany in that same year.

The U.S. revolution in herbal medicine is consumer driven. Studies of this social phenomenon have been done at esteemed places such as the Harvard University School of Medicine. In 1993 David Eisenberg, M.D., and his colleagues at Harvard reported in the *New England Journal of Medicine* that over one-third of Americans surveyed were seeking treatment more often from alternative medicine practitioners than from internists, pediatricians, primary care, and other conventional physicians.[1] These people complained particularly about modern medicine's reflexlike prescription of drugs and were seeking more natural medicines that focused on the patient as a whole. The study reported that in 1990 Americans paid over ten billion dollars from their own pockets for alternative treatments such as herbal medicine and homeopathy (a system for treating disease based on the administration of minute doses of a substance that in massive amounts produces symptoms in healthy individuals similar to those of the disease itself; see pages 135–138).

A 1997 national survey conducted by *Prevention Magazine* reported that approximately one-third (32 percent) of adult Americans frequently use herbal medicines. About sixty million Americans each spent an average of fifty-four dollars on herbal remedies in 1996. Pharmacy sales of herbal dietary supplements are increasing more rapidly than sales of any other products. Herbal remedies are the second fastest growing sales category. The survey showed that a majority of these consumers found the herbal products better than, or just as good as, synthetic drugs.

People are seeking herbal medicines in part because they are afraid of the drugs used in conventional medicine. Pharmaceuticals, both prescription and over-the-counter drugs, are responsible for over 150,000 deaths in the United States each year. A study in the *Journal of the American Medical Association* reported that three of every one thousand people who are hospitalized die as a result of the pharmaceuticals they are given.

Synthetic drugs can be toxic and are frequently accompanied by unpleasant side effects. Often one drug is used to treat the side effects of another! As a result, people have come to seek safer, gentler, more natural herbal treatments. The rising cost of pharmaceuticals compared with the price of herbs has also become a factor. For example, the daily cost of three *Hypericum* tablets is about sixty cents compared with a few dollars for two synthetic antidepressant tablets. Pharmaceuticals have become a multibillion-dollar international industry with huge profits, while many people cannot afford their pharmacy bills. In today's managed care environment, the cost savings of herbal medicines, as compared to synthetic drugs, makes them ever more attractive.

Once considered exotic, herbal medicine is now moving into the mainstream because of increasing public interest in natural health care. This consumer-driven revolution is demanding change from modern medicine. In September 1997, Cedars-Sinai Medical Center of Los Angeles opened a Complementary Medicine Program, which included making herbal medicine available to its patients. A rapidly growing number of U.S. health care clinics are offering an integrative approach, incorporating both modern and herbal medicines. Dozens of medical schools across the country are now adding complementary medicine courses to their curriculum so that future physicians can offer natural healing and herbal medicine to patients.

In addition, the science supporting herbal medicine has advanced. Medical and laboratory studies are creating a new level of acceptance of herbal medicine among health professionals. Increasingly, insurance companies and health maintenance organizations (HMOs) are waking up to this growing trend and offering coverage for natural treatments.

Media coverage of natural health care has increased tremendously in recent years. For example, Bill Moyers' and

Andrew Weil's public television specials brought many former skeptics into natural food stores to take a closer look at herbal medicine. Today there are best-selling books on herbal medicines, including *Miracle Cures* by Jean Carper (HarperCollins, 1997), *Spontaneous Healing* by Andrew Weil (Knopf, 1995), and my previous book *Hypericum (St.-John's-Wort) and Depression* (Prelude Press, 1996). The emphasis on disease care in the United States is shifting to incorporate self-care (including prevention) and self-education about health, fitness, and nutrition. Herbal medicine fits naturally into this revolution.

THE RETURN TO
NATURE'S PHARMACY

Herbal remedies work in one respect like pharmaceutical drugs, through active biochemical compounds. Indeed, the remarkable renaissance of interest in these natural substances is due in part to the fact that modern researchers are achieving consistent and reproducible results in clinical and laboratory studies using standardized botanical extracts.

Almost one-third of prescribed medicines are obtained from plants or are synthesized versions of biochemicals originally found in botanicals. For example, aspirin originates from the bark of the white willow tree, digitalis from the foxglove plant, and penicillin from a mold (a primitive plant form). Yet medical science mistakenly assumed that a single isolated compound was always better than the complex mixture of substances in the plant itself. Isolated or synthetic drugs are often more toxic and have fewer safeguards than their natural sources. Indeed, the whole herb may be more effective than isolated pharmaceutical compounds. The whole of a plant's active substances is greater than the sum of its individual constituents because the active biochemicals within exist in natural ratios, which human genes have experienced and adapted to in the course of evolution.

Consumers and physicians accustomed to the instant relief of synthetic tranquilizers and sleeping pills sometimes become impatient with herbal medicines. While the initial effect of an herb may be less dramatic, the healing it facilitates can be deeper and more lasting. Each medicinal herb has its own creative intelligence, a unique constellation of healing energy. Human genes have evolved alongside these natural chemicals but have not been exposed to synthetic drugs until modern times. This is one reason why in many cases herbs are more effective and gentler than drugs, with far fewer, if any, side effects.

ECHINACEA: THE PURPLE DAISY

A decline in the use of herbal medicines in this country began with the introduction of antibiotics in the 1940s. For most of the last fifty years, American medicine has focused on synthesizing substances to "conquer" disease and disease-causing organisms, without regard for natural consequences. The overuse of antibiotics has created "superbacteria"—antibiotic-resistant strains of *Staphylococcus, Streptococcus, Gonorrhea,* and others.

A 1997 study reported in the *Journal of the American Medical Association* found that physicians inappropriately prescribe antibiotics for viral infections 70 percent of the time, even though they know that antibiotics are not effective against viral infections. Doctors wrote twelve million prescriptions in 1992 for antibiotics to treat colds, bronchitis, and other respiratory infections against which these drugs are useless. Researchers concluded that physicians were prescribing antibiotics because they were yielding to what they perceived to be their patients' expectations.

Thirty-two double-blind, placebo-controlled studies on the herb *Echinacea* suggest that this member of the daisy family can combat colds and the flu through its virus-fighting activity and as a natural immune system enhancer. Paradoxically, it initially took European research to validate this remarkable American Indian herb, native to the Great Plains of the United States. *Echinacea* does not create strains of bacteria that become resistant to it, as antibiotics do. Also, *Echinacea* is much less expensive than antibiotics.

If you are trying to fight off a cold or flu, it is best to use a standardized concentration of *Echinacea* and follow the dosage instructions on the label. Also, check the label to make sure the product is standardized for echinacoside, the active compound, and that it contains only *Echinacea purpurea* and *Echinacea angustifolia*. *Echinacea* must be taken at the first sign of a cold or flu and taken for one week to be effective. If you are allergic to daisies, *Echinacea* may trigger watery eyes. Other than this rare, mild allergic reaction, *Echinacea* is so safe that pediatricians recommend it for six-month-old babies to fight viral respiratory infections. In 1996 Americans spent eighty million dollars on *Echinacea* products, up 25 percent from the previous year.

Echinacea is just one example of natural remedies that are safer, milder, and sometimes more effective than their pharmaceutical counterparts. Similarly, as I shall describe, there are many effective, safe, and inexpensive alternatives to the millions of prescriptions for tranquilizers and sleeping pills written by physicians.

10

Using Herbs Safely and Appropriately

Anxiety, stress, and insomnia are some of the most troublesome problems to treat with conventional medicine. The drugs used have many side effects, and most are habit-forming. Natural remedies provide safe alternatives and are becoming the first treatment choice.

—ROB MCCALEB,
HERB RESEARCH FOUNDATION

When reading the label on an herbal preparation, keep in mind that manufacturers are prevented by current law from stating that herbs can help treat or prevent diseases or symptoms. According to the 1994 Dietary Supplement Health and Education Act (DSHEA), herbs are considered supplements, not drugs. Manufacturers are able to claim that their products can enhance general well-being or that they can support or help improve body functions, such as circulation or digestion, so long as the claim is supported by scientific evidence.

A few unscrupulous companies are making inappropriate claims regarding poor-quality or unproven herbal products that the DSHEA had made it difficult for the Food and Drug Administration (FDA) to regulate. A 1997 presidential commission on dietary supplements proposed that a new set of regulations be instituted to ensure good manufacturing practices for herbal medicines and to help weed out unethical companies. Consumers are urged to buy products only from reputable manufacturers. To find out which companies are the most respected, check with your physician, health food store, or pharmacy.

The ideal policy for medicinal herbs in the United States would be to adopt the German standard for sanctioning herbs as drugs: absolute proof of safety and reasonable proof of efficacy (see "Germany's Commission E," below). This would allow the best medically proven herbs to be approved as over-the-counter (OTC) drugs. The American Herbal Products Association, the Utah Natural Products Alliance, the European-American Phytomedicines Coalition, the National Nutritional Foods Association, and the Council for Responsible Nutrition are all lobbying for OTC drug status for herbal medicines. In Germany and in much of Europe, OTC herbs are already regulated as drugs, ensuring that standards of quality are high.

In any case, it is important to educate yourself about any herbal remedy or synthetic drug that you consider taking. Don't use any substance without being familiar with therapeutic indications, dosages, side effects, and contraindications (factors that render the administration of a drug or herb inadvisable). Do not self-diagnose for potentially serious medical conditions or use a clerk at a health food store as a surrogate doctor or pharmacist. It is always best to consult a physician for a diagnostic checkup and a discussion of therapeutic options.

In addition to the herbal medicines for healing anxiety and stress discussed in this book, there are other herbs that have been scientifically studied and proven effective to treat many diseases and promote health. Based on scientific studies from around the world, the following herbs are recommended for the conditions listed. Adequate medical scrutiny has shown that they consistently offer therapeutic value, efficacy, and safety.

Herb: Saw palmetto berry
Condition: Benign prostatic hyperplasia
Standardization: 85–95% fatty acids and sterols

Herb: Garlic
Condition: High cholesterol; viral, fungal, bacterial conditions
Standardization: 3.4% alliin

Herb: *Pygeum Africanum*
Condition: Benign prostatic hyperplasia
Standardization: 13% total sterols

Herb: Feverfew
Condition: Migraine headaches
Standardization: 0.6% parthenolide

Herb: Cranberry
Condition: Urinary tract infection
Standardization: 5% anthocyanidins, 30% organic acids, 20% arbutin

Herb: Black cohosh
Condition: Menopausal symptoms
Standardization: 1 mg of triterpene glycosides calculated as 27-deoxyactein

Herb: Grape seed
Condition: Inflammation, athrosclerosis, bruising, oxidation, vascular disease, varicose veins
Standardization: 95% procyanidolic oligomers

Herb: Bilberry
Condition: Cataracts, myopia, night blindness, diabetic retinopathy, macular degeneration
Standardization: 25% anthocyanosides calculated as anthocyanidins

Herb: Ginger
Condition: Nausea, motion sickness
Standardization: 20% pungent compounds, calculated as 6-gingerol and 6-shogaol

If you already have a known medical disease or take prescription drugs, discuss with your doctor whether herbs are safe for you. Do not discontinue medically approved conventional treatments without medical supervision. If you have any unusual side effects from an herb, stop taking it and call your physician immediately.

If you are pregnant, consult with your obstetrician or other health care provider before taking any herb. Some herbs contain substances that can cause a miscarriage or premature labor or damage the fetus. Little research has been done on using herbs during pregnancy or breast-feeding, so caution is strongly recommended.

Just because an herb is natural doesn't mean it is always safe. Ephedra, or *mahuang*, for example, should be avoided by anyone with anxiety, hypertension, diabetes, glaucoma, or elevated thyroid. Comfrey and coltsfoot contain toxins that can damage the liver. Some plants, like water hemlock and belladonna, can be deadly and are therefore prohibited by the FDA.

No substance is perfectly safe. Among the few people who have become ill after taking medicinal herbs, some had the mistaken notion that if something is natural, it is safe in any dosage. Others may have unusual allergic reactions to herbs that are safe for most people, just as some people have food allergies. Although side effects are few and generally mild, you should consider them carefully before taking any herb and take only the recommended dosage.

The herbal remedies recommended in this book enjoy an excellent safety record over thousands of years of folk medicine. These herbs generally are less toxic and have fewer side effects than their synthetic counterparts. The last decade has seen an explosion of scientific research on these herbal medicines, including their therapeutic uses, contraindications, dosage recommendations, and other pertinent safety considerations.

GERMANY'S COMMISSION E

Germany is the world's role model for high standards in herbal medicine. Much of the revolutionary scientific research on the effectiveness of medicinal herbs comes from Germany, a country with a continuous, highly respected tradition of herbal medicine. German physicians are trained in the use of these natural remedies while they are in medical school, and about 80 percent prescribe herbal medicines in their practices. In contrast, the United States has had a broken tradition of herb use because of social and economic factors. Unrealistic federal regulations have hampered research on herbal remedies by making such research unprofitable for American pharmaceutical companies. To get FDA approval of a natural remedy as a new drug can cost tens of millions of dollars and take seven or more years. And because a plant cannot be patented in the United States, there is little economic incentive for American companies to investigate and develop a botanical medicine as a new pharmaceutical drug.

In Germany, herbal medicines are approved as OTC drugs by a governmental agency similar to our FDA. Germany's Commission E is a special scientific committee of the *Bundesgesundheitsamt* (Federal Department of Health) that has actively collected research data on herbal medicines, evaluating their effectiveness and safety. The results are published as monographs, which are considered among the top scientific compendiums on herbs in the world. Commission E consists of a panel of consumers and experts including physicians, pharmacologists, toxicologists, and pharmaceutical industry representatives specializing in herbal medicine. The commission reviews studies of animal and pharmacological research, human clinical trials, medical practice, and quality control investigations of herbal cultivation and manufacturing.

Since 1978 Commission E has published 410 monographs covering 324 individual herbs and various herbal combinations. Each monograph describes the herb's effectiveness, side effects, contraindications, and proper therapeutic dosage. Each monograph includes a positive or negative assessment. For an herb to gain Commission E approval, it must show strong evidence of safety and a reasonable assurance of effectiveness. The labeling of herbal products for OTC use is based on the commission's assessment and includes a caution when a specific herb's benefits may not be proven. The American Botanical Council, under the direction of Mark Blumenthal, in 1997 published an English translation of the German Commission E monographs.

STANDARDIZED HERBAL PRODUCTS

All natural products are not created equal. Some cost more, and some are always discounted. However, price tags provide no information about the health benefits contained inside a package. If price is the sole criterion by which a product is purchased, the goal of achieving good health will probably not be attained. There's more to selecting an herbal product than price and knowing what condition it can help. Quality is essential. It is not the herb that provides the benefit but the active ingredients found in the herb. It is not the name on the label that ensures effective results but the quality and concentration of the active ingredients found in the herb. Because there is so much disparity among the multitude of products available, consumers should make their selections carefully.

The best way to ensure quality is to buy herbal products that are standardized. A standardized herbal product provides specific concentrations of an herb's active ingredients dose after dose. Standardization guarantees consistency in herbal products for a predictable effect.[1]

Standardization is a manufacturing process that ensures that an herbal product contains agreed-upon levels of certain chemicals or compounds believed to be active ingredients of that herb or reliable markers for the presence of adequate amounts of herb in the product. Standardization is not a measure of the strength or potency of the herbal product, but it guarantees that it contains a consistent amount of the chosen compounds.

The reason for standardization is to assure consistency of therapeutic effect. Nonstandardized extracts may also be effective, but since most modern clinical research is performed using standardized extracts, less evidence exists to support the use of nonstandardized extracts. In addition, some herbal products are not standardized, because researchers have not yet identified which active ingredients are reliable markers for those plants.

The worldwide research performed on herbs does not ensure results unless standardization information is understood and used. For instance, there are many grades and qualities of the herb sold under the name of *Hypericum* (Saint-John's-wort), and not all of these products are effective. The landmark studies on *Hypericum* for the treatment of depression call for the herb to be standardized at 0.3 percent hypericin. Using a Saint-John's-wort product containing anything less than 0.3 percent hypericin will not guarantee results. On the other hand, when the level of potency matches the medical studies, the health benefits are uniform.

Choose products from a reputable manufacturer. Producing good natural products can be challenging because the quality of herbs and plants used varies greatly as a result of climate, growing conditions, and conditions of harvesting and storing. These variables can dramatically affect the nutritional and therapeutic benefits of the final product. Only the most advanced manufacturers combine nature and technology to create products that contain research-grade ingredients in amounts that have been scientifically validated. The best manufacturers have on-site laboratories, closely monitor processes, and standardize to ensure consistent potency from batch to batch. Enzymatic Therapy, Nature's Herbs, and Nature's Way are examples of leading herbal manufacturers whose quality products are found at fine health food stores. Sunsource and Murdock-Madaus-Schwabe, also dedicated to high-quality products, are distributed solely to pharmacies, supermarkets, and discount stores nationwide.

Large manufacturers in Europe and the United States are increasingly adhering to quality control methods that ensure that the herbal product you purchase is consistently pure and safe. Modern herb extraction processes integrate the age-old knowledge of folk remedies with scientific standards. Techniques of cultivation, drying, storage, grinding, extraction, and concentration are carefully controlled and tested to make sure that the final capsules, tablets, or liquid preparations are of consistent quality.

Some herbs are so mild in their effects that it is impractical to try to consume enough of the plants in bulk form or tablets to obtain their benefits. Therefore an extract is made, which concentrates the active ingredients by mixing the crude herb (the flowers, leaves, or roots) with alcohol or another solvent. A solid residue remains when all of the solvent is evaporated off. This solid extract, available in powdered form in either capsules or tablets, represents the most concentrated form of an herbal medicine. Herbal teas, which use water as the solvent, are relatively weak. These may be more suitable for children, elderly people, and others who are especially sensitive to the effects of herbs.

II

Herbal Medicines or Synthetic Drugs for Anxiety?

If you are faced with the prospect of taking drugs to treat a health problem, you will want to know if there are any natural agents you may use instead.
—ANDREW WEIL, M.D.

Each year Americans take billions of doses of benzodiazepines for anxiety and insomnia. Common benzodiazepine tranquilizers include Valium (diazepam), Xanax (alprazolam), Ativan (lorazepam), Tranxene (clorazepate), and Klonopin (clonazepam). Common benzodiazepine sleeping pills include Dalmane (flurazepam), Restoril (temazepam), Halcion (triazolam), and Serax (oxazepam). These are addictive and can produce drowsiness, impaired coordination, poor concentration, memory impairment, and amnesia. Narcotics, birth control pills, Inderal (propranolol), and other sedatives can make such side effects even worse. Regular benzodiazepine use can also exacerbate depression.

Synthetic tranquilizers should only be prescribed for moderate to severe anxiety or panic disorder. But because they are addictive, they should never be used for longer than two to three weeks. Use for a longer period of time can cause physical and psychological dependence. People susceptible to abusing alcohol or drugs can become addicted to benzodiazepines after a single dose. Alcohol should not be consumed when taking benzodiazepines, because their interaction can depress both breathing and blood pressure, possibly causing a coma or death. Abrupt discontinuation of benzodiazepines taken for more than three weeks can also cause significant withdrawal symptoms. Among these are anxiety, insomnia, and panic attacks, symptoms that may have led the person to take these drugs in the first place! Benzodiazepine treatment therefore has a high relapse rate.

If used to treat insomnia, benzodiazepines can cause abnormal sleeping patterns and a morning hangover. Synthetic drugs do not produce natural sleep; they chemically knock you out. Despite regulatory and professional cautions, about 20 percent of chronic insomniacs take these addictive agents nightly for years. As with benzodiazepine tranquilizers, abrupt discontinuation of these sedatives often causes rebound insomnia, the condition these pills are meant to alleviate.

ANTIDEPRESSANTS
TO ALLEVIATE ANXIETY

When anxiety is moderate to severe or herbal medicines are ineffective, synthetic antidepressants may be necessary for brief periods until the antidepressants start to work. Antidepressants can be effective for 60 to 80 percent of those with panic attacks or other anxiety disorders. The drugs proven to be most effective in treating obsessive-compulsive disorder (OCD) are four antidepressants—Anafranil (clomipramine), Luvox (fluvox), Prozac (fluoxetine), and Zoloft (sertraline). There has been no research on herbal treatment for OCD. There are roughly a dozen antidepressants from which to choose if synthetic antidepressants are prescribed. None are addictive or habit-forming.

Antidepressant medications are usually taken for two to three weeks before benefits are derived. During this time, patience and perseverance are essential. Some patients decide the medication doesn't work after a few days or weeks and discontinue it. Others experience side effects and stop without telling their doctor. Either response is a mistake.

Communicate any side effects to your doctor. If the problem is especially troublesome, call at once; don't wait until your next appointment. Your doctor may wish to prescribe a different antidepressant, but if your doctor suggests continuing with the medication as prescribed, please consider doing so. Most side effects disappear within two to three weeks.

Because of the length of time it takes to see the results from taking antidepressants, it may take a while for you and your doctor to arrive at the proper medication and dosage. Be patient with the process. During the initial phase of treatment, you may require more frequent consultations with your doctor. Do not change your medication or dosage on your own. If selective serotonin reuptake inhibitors (SSRIs) are discontinued too abruptly, the result can be serotonin withdrawal syndrome, with flulike symptoms. A gradual dose reduction of SSRIs is necessary.

SSRIs, such as Prozac (fluoxetine) and Effexor (venlafaxine), can sometimes *cause* nervousness, agitation, insomnia, palpitations, sweating, and sexual dysfunction. These side effects can easily be mistaken for symptoms of anxiety, the disorder these medicines are attempting to treat. If the side effects are severe, you and your doctor may decide to lower the dosage or discontinue the drug and try a different medication.

Do not take any additional drugs—OTC, prescription, or recreational—without first consulting your health care provider. Drugs that when taken alone are relatively harmless can become dangerous, even deadly, when taken with some antidepressants.

HERBS AS A FIRST-LINE TREATMENT FOR ANXIETY

The first rule of medicine is *Primum non nocere*, which means "Above all, do no harm." Asclepios of Thessaly, a great physician of antiquity, gave the following advice for the use of medicines: "First the word, then the plant." Three thousand years later R. F. Weiss, M.D., updated this principle as follows: "First the word, then the plant drug, next the major synthetic chemotherapeutic agent."[1]

If patients persist in complaints to their doctors about stress and anxiety, they can walk out of the office with a prescription for the Valium-like tranquilizers or sleeping pills. Overprescription of benzodiazepine tranquilizers and sleeping pills has reached epidemic proportions. These drugs are often abused because, until now, most doctors and patients were unaware of herbal alternatives. Mild anxiety, stress, and insomnia may require neither herbs nor synthetic drugs. Natural self-healing techniques alone can suffice (see Part 3). When a medicinal agent is needed, however, herbal remedies deserve to be considered before synthetic drugs because of their relative safety and fewer side effects, as well as their effectiveness.

HEALING ANXIETY
WITH HERBS CHECKLIST

After you and your doctor have ruled out an anxiety disorder or any other medical or psychiatric illness, the herbal medicines discussed in Part 2 can be used to heal the following signs and symptoms of anxiety and stress and anxiety (mentioned here for those who may have skipped Part 1), *provided they are mild to moderate*:

- Nervousness
- Trembling, shaking
- Rapid heartbeat
- Cold, clammy hands
- Indigestion, knot in the stomach
- Dizziness, faintness, light-headedness
- Hyperventilation
- Work strain
- Numbness and tingling sensations
- Excessive worry
- Insomnia, nightmares
- Muscular aches and pains
- Tension headaches
- Fatigue
- Overeating
- Premenstrual tension
- Persistent shyness
- Fear of flying and other simple phobias
- Chronic irritability
- Difficulty concentrating
- Performance anxiety
- Excessive sweating
- Chills or hot flashes
- Hyperactivity

- Attention deficit
- Nicotine withdrawal
- Depression
- Fears of sexual performance
- Memory difficulties
- "Hurry dis-ease," feeling constantly impatient and under pressure
- Clenched teeth, bruxism
- Feeling chronically insecure, unsafe
- Lack of sexual energy and vitality
- Inability to relax, mind keeps racing
- Obsession with the past or fear of the future
- Difficulty unwinding without alcohol

A commitment to the natural self-healing program (Part 3), without the use of medicinal herbs or synthetic drugs, may suffice if symptoms of anxiety are few and mild. If you have a number of moderate symptoms, medicinal herbs along with the tools and techniques of the natural self-healing program will probably be necessary. Again, if your symptoms are moderate to severe at this time, don't despair. Pharmaceutical medicines or psychotherapy can be very effective in consultation with a supportive health professional to launch you on your way to natural self-healing. You and your doctor can periodically reevaluate when a switch to herbal medicines would be appropriate.

Herbal remedies can be a first-line treatment for many millions of people suffering from mild to moderate anxiety. Kava should be considered for anxiety (see chapter 12) and valerian as a sleep aid (see pages 91–94) before prescribing tranquilizers or sleeping pills. *Hypericum*, an antidepressant, can also help to reduce anxiety (see chapter 13).

You and your physician should discuss fully whether herbal medicines or synthetic drugs are appropriate for your condition and also what the potential benefits, side effects, risks, and length of treatment might be. If your doctor is not familiar with prescribing herbs for anxiety and refuses to become informed, ask for a referral to a naturopathic or osteopathic physician, herbalist, or chiropractor who has this knowledge (see Appendix C). It is time for health professionals to wake up and smell the herbs!

Sometimes the herbal remedy initially chosen does not produce the desired result. Don't give up. Often the second or third alternative will produce the desired benefit. This may be due to subtle differences in individual needs. Some herbs work right away; others may take three to four weeks to exert their benefits. Although the herbal medicines used to treat anxiety and insomnia are not addicting, you should be under a doctor's care.

Many patients who have been taking pharmaceutical tranquilizers and sleeping pills have difficulty discontinuing these drugs. Rapid withdrawal from benzodiazepines can cause severe or even dangerous symptoms. While herbs can support this process, tapering off and discontinuing these drugs can be challenging, and should be done under careful medical supervision.

12

Kava—the Natural Tranquilizer

Kava may one day replace benzodiaze-pines in the pharmacological treatment of anxiety.
—MICHAEL T. MURRAY, N.D.,
NATURAL ALTERNATIVES TO PROZAC

Kava kava, or simply kava, is rapidly becoming an herbal superstar. Its calming effects have generated increasing scientific interest because synthetic tranquilizers are generally not suitable for longer than three weeks. Whereas benzodiazepine tranquilizers can be addictive, impair memory, and worsen a depression, kava improves mental functioning and mood and is not addictive.

Kava pills come in different strengths, usually from 100 to 250 mg, and the percentage of kavalactones (the active chemicals in kava) in the extract can vary from 30 to 70 percent. The dosage used in most clinical studies for anxiety is three daily 100-mg doses of kava extract standardized to 70-percent kavalactone content, which research has shown can be as effective as the benzodiazepine drug Serax (oxazepam),

15 mg daily. A 70-percent kava extract is not yet commercially available in the United States.

Enzymatic Therapy has a 150-mg capsule of a 55-percent kava extract, which would contain 82.5 mg of kavalactones. A 100-mg capsule of 70-percent kava extract would equal 70 mg of kavalactones (.70 x 100). A 250-mg capsule of 30-percent extract would contain 75 mg of kavalactones (.30 x 250). It is best to begin with a total daily dosage of 70 to 85 mg of kavalactones, taken in the evening. Stay on one capsule if it effectively reduces anxiety. If it is not enough, you can add a second pill in the morning. Remain on this twice daily dosage for at least a week. If you still feel tense or fearful after that, you can add a third capsule in the middle of the day. When you consistently feel more relaxed, you can gradually decrease your dosage by one pill every few days.

Consuming kava on a daily basis is not recommended for longer than twenty-five weeks (four to six months). When used in small amounts on an occasional basis, it can be used longer, if necessary. If 70 to 85 mg of kavalactones three times a day is not effective for your anxiety, see your doctor for a reevaluation to see if taking more kava is indicated or if you may require a prescription drug.

Unless you are under medical supervision, do not combine kava with benzodiazepine tranquilizers. In 1996 Dr. Y. N. Singh reported in a letter to the *Annals of Internal Medicine* that a patient became disoriented and lethargic after combining Xanax (alprazolam) and kava, requiring brief hospitalization. This case suggests that kava can potentiate the sedative effect of benzodiazepines. If you are taking a synthetic tranquilizer, you should be gradually withdrawn from it under medical supervision before beginning kava.

Kava (*Piper methysticum*) is a member of the pepper tree family, native to Fiji, Samoa, and other South Pacific islands, where it was traditionally consumed by Polynesian chieftains during ceremonial rites. A description of kava's effects was written in 1777 by George Forster, a naturalist aboard Captain James Cook's ship. Cook and his crew introduced kava to the Western world following this South Pacific voyage. Today the thick, knotty kava root is cultivated throughout the South Pacific islands for local consumption as a beverage and to export for processing as a natural tranquilizer. The active chemicals, the kavalactones, are concentrated in the root, which is harvested at three to four years of age for optimal potency.

English, German, Swiss, and other European health boards have approved kava for the treatment of anxiety and insomnia. Research studies have demonstrated that kava can relieve a wide range of anxiety symptoms. Although researchers are not yet sure exactly how kava works, some researchers theorize that it has a direct soothing action on an overactive amygdala, the brain's alarm center, thereby both relieving anxiety and elevating mood. Kava does not appear to lose its benefits over time and does not impair memory.

In a 1996 randomized, placebo-controlled, double-blind study, two groups of 29 patients with anxiety syndromes were treated with 100 mg of kava extract standardized to 70-percent kavalactones three times a day for four weeks. The symptoms of anxiety were significantly reduced in patients taking kava as compared to placebo. No adverse reactions were observed in the kava group.

In a 1997 multicenter, randomized, placebo-controlled study reported by Drs. Volz and Kieser in the journal *Pharmacopsychiatry*, a total of 101 outpatients were given one capsule of a kava extract containing 70 mg of kavalactones or placebo three times daily. In this twenty-five-week study, all the patients suffered from moderate to severe anxiety, including agoraphobia, generalized anxiety disorder, specific phobia, and social phobia. The results showed that the short- and long-term effectiveness of kava was superior to that of placebo. After twenty-four weeks, over half of the kava group were rated as "very improved": anxiety, fear, tension, and insomnia decreased steadily with treatment. Kava was well tolerated, and adverse reactions were mild and rare. The researchers concluded that kava was a treatment alternative to both benzodiazepines and synthetic antidepressants for anxiety disorders.

At ten times the recommended dosage, consumed for many months, some heavy drinkers of kava root in the Polynesian islands have developed a scaly eruption or yellowing of the skin associated with muscle spasms, biochemical abnormalities, vision disturbances, and even shortness of breath. Such skin problems associated with kava abuse have not been reported in the United States or Europe. These disturbances go away quickly when kava is discontinued. Large intake of kava is unnecessary and strongly discouraged. At the recommended therapeutic levels, no such side effects have been reported.

Kava should not be taken by people suffering from Parkinson's disease, because it might worsen muscular weakness and twitching. A few cases of an allergic reaction to kava have been reported. Kava should also not be taken after ingesting alcohol or mixed with pharmaceutical antidepressants, benzodiazepine tranquilizers, or sleeping pills. Care should be taken when driving or operating machinery. People who are elderly or medically ill should take smaller doses of kava and only under a doctor's supervision. Kava is not recommended during pregnancy or breast-feeding or for severe anxiety disorders and depression.

Kava reduces anxiety without causing the lethargy, diminished concentration, and fuzziness so often associated with synthetic tranquilizers. Though caution is always indicated, people who are taking appropriate doses of kava can generally drive an automobile or focus on work without experiencing any sedation. With the growing availability of high-quality kava products, this natural tranquilizer could soon become a first-line treatment for mild to moderate anxiety.

13

Healing Anxiety with *Hypericum* (Saint-John's-Wort)

Hypericum is an absolutely amazing medical discovery, a simple herb that could change the lives of millions of Americans.
—BARBARA WALTERS,
ABC TV's *20/20*

Hypericum perforatum, commonly known as Saint-John's-wort (*wort* means "plant"), is a perennial plant with bright yellow flowers that start to bloom annually around June 20, Saint John's birthday. *Hypericum* was recommended by Hippocrates for "nervous unrest." It has a 2400-year history of folk use for anxiety, sleep disturbances, and worry. Modern medical research has shown that *Hypericum* can be as effective as prescription antidepressants for mild to moderate depression.[1] However, unlike prescription antidepressants, *Hypericum*'s side effects are few and mild. Also, *Hypericum* costs considerably less and is available without a prescription, making it one of the most accessible herbal medicines. *Hyper-*

icum is now the number one antidepressant, natural or synthetic, prescribed by German physicians. In Germany, *Hypericum* accounts for over 50 percent of the antidepressant market, while Prozac is down to 2 percent.

In addition to *Hypericum*'s mood-elevating properties, Germany's Commission E has approved this remarkable herb for the treatment of anxiety and sleep disorders. *Hypericum* cannot be taken as a tranquillizer to acutely relieve anxiety. Its capacity to reduce anxiety depends upon its antidepressant effect, which can take a few weeks to kick in. In two clinical studies, *Hypericum* demonstrated antianxiety effects comparable to those of Valium (diazepam). Yet *Hypericum* is not addictive and does not impair cognitive functions.

How does this herb work its wonders? *Hypericum* extract contains numerous active compounds that together create the antidepressant and antianxiety effects. *Hypericum* is the first known substance to enhance three key neurotransmitters— serotonin, norepinephrine, and dopamine. Preliminary research suggests that this remarkable herb also lowers levels of the stress hormone cortisol and enhances the activity of gamma-aminobutyric acid (GABA), a naturally occurring tranquilizer in the brain. It is a very mild, clinically insignificant monoamine oxidase (MAO) inhibitor.

Contrary to the warnings in some outdated reports, it is not necessary when taking *Hypericum* to adhere to the dietary restrictions that are required when taking MAO inhibitor drugs. However, any selective serotonin reuptake inhibitor (SSRI), including *Hypericum*, should not be combined with a MAO inhibitor antidepressant such as Nardil (phenelzine) or Parnate (tranylcypromine). This combination can produce a dangerous rise in blood pressure or hypertensive crisis, along with severe anxiety, fever, muscle tension, and confusion. After stopping a MAO inhibitor, one should wait at least four weeks before taking other antidepressants, including *Hypericum*.

If you are being treated successfully with prescription antidepressants for anxiety or depression with minimal side effects and low cost, there may be no need to switch to *Hypericum*. Clinical research on switching from prescription antidepressants to *Hypericum* is needed. If you are currently taking synthetic antidepressants and you and your doctor decide to switch to *Hypericum* extract, certain safeguards must be respected.

Clinical experience suggests that the most effective way to make the transition from a synthetic SSRI to *Hypericum* is to gradually reduce the dosage of the prescription antidepressant while slowly, over a couple of weeks, building up to a dosage of *Hypericum* extract of 300 mg three times daily. You and your doctor must at the same time be careful to avoid the medical condition known as serotonin syndrome, the result of having too much of the serotonin neurotransmitter, which is the opposite of what happens in anxiety and depression. The symptoms can include sweating, agitation, lethargy, confusion, tremor, and muscle spasms. If such symptoms occur, consult your physician immediately. Either the synthetic SSRI or the *Hypericum* extract must be reduced until these symptoms abate.

If all is well once the *Hypericum* is added, wait another few weeks before discontinuing the synthetic SSRI, again under medical supervision. The rebound effect of stopping prescription antidepressants too abruptly can be severe. A serotonin withdrawal syndrome has been described, consisting of flulike symptoms, when synthetic SSRIs are too abruptly stopped.

There may be a few bumps in the transition from a synthetic antidepressant to *Hypericum*, so stay in close touch with your doctor. Also, remember that for some people *Hypericum* does not work as well as a prescription antidepressant. At present, *Hypericum* should only be considered for anxiety that is mild to moderate, and not for an anxiety disorder. Also, please remember that natural self-healing (see Part 3) and cognitive-behavioral psychotherapy (see page 221) can also be important to your healing.

Saint-John's-wort has an exceptional safety record over centuries of folk medicine. In contrast to synthetic antidepressants, there have been no reports of *Hypericum*-related deaths. Drug monitoring studies on over 7000 patients and twenty-seven double-blind research studies confirm its safety. The extensive use of *Hypericum* by millions of people has not resulted in reports of serious side effects, even from overdose.

The potential for phototoxicity, a hypersensitivity to sunlight, should be kept in mind if one spends time in the sun or if one is taking other photosensitizing drugs such as chlorpromazine and tetracycline. While severe photosensitivity reactions have not been well documented in humans (there are reports on sheep grazing on very large quantities of Saint-John's-wort while exposed to the sun), people with fair skin should use added sun protection while they are taking this herb.

Dr. Klaus Linde and colleagues thoroughly reviewed all of the studies reported in the medical literature on the effectiveness and safety of *Hypericum*. Their results were published in the August 3, 1996 issue of the *British Medical Journal*. Based on data from 1008 patients in only those studies deemed most scientifically sound, the results showed that *Hypericum* extracts were indeed more effective than placebo in the treatment of mild to moderately severe depression. In addition, six comparison studies found that *Hypericum* was as effective as synthetic antidepressants but with fewer side effects. These studies reported that 10.8 percent of the patients had side effects with *Hypericum* (gastrointestinal irritation, dizziness, dry mouth, and a few mild allergic reactions), while 35.9 percent reported side effects from prescription antidepressants. The *British Medical Journal* report emphasized that the side effects of *Hypericum* were "rare and mild." Less than 5 percent of people stop taking *Hypericum* because of side effects.

In a major study by Drs. Woelk *et al.* reported in the *Journal of Geriatric Psychiatry and Neurology* in October 1994, 3250 patients were treated with 300 mg *Hypericum* extract three times daily by 633 physicians. Eight typical complaints heard in general practice were recorded: depression, gastrointestinal symptoms, restlessness, difficulty initiating sleep, difficulty falling asleep, headaches, cardiac symptoms, and sweating. About 80 percent of the patients felt improved after four weeks, as measured by medical and patient evaluations. Side effects were seen in only 2.4 percent of subjects.

The typical dosage of *Hypericum*, based on the majority of medical studies, is 300 mg of *Hypericum* extract standardized to 0.3-percent hypericin three times a day. If nausea or gastrointestinal distress is a problem, take it with each meal—breakfast, lunch, and dinner—though it is not known to what extent food affects absorption. Sometimes a reduction of the dosage to 300 mg once or twice daily is called for while the body adjusts.

Although no cases of problems during pregnancy and lactation have been reported after decades of extensive use in Germany, *Hypericum* cannot as yet be recommended during pregnancy because of insufficient research data. The natural antidepressants contained in *Hypericum* are obtained through alcohol extraction. This is why a tea made from Saint-John's-wort (i.e., water extraction) is not as effective. Only 10 to 20 percent of the total hypericin content is dissolved into tea. You would have to drink *Hypericum* tea throughout the day to obtain significant benefits.

Hypericum might be an alternative in the treatment of severe, recurrent depression. In a 1997 randomized, double-blind study by Dr. Vorbach and colleagues published in *Phar-*

macopsychiatry, 209 patients with severe, recurrent depression (but with no psychotic or delusional symptoms) were treated for six weeks with 600 mg of *Hypericum* extract (standardized to 0.3-percent hypericin) three times a day. This high-dose treatment (1800 mg daily of *Hypericum* is double the usual dosage) proved equal to treatment with a full dose of Tofranil (imipramine) (50 mg three times daily), but even at this higher dosage *Hypericum* showed considerably less side effects. Of course, you should not consider going up to 1800 mg daily without intensive medical supervision. More studies on treating severe depression with *Hypericum* are needed.

Hypericum's effectiveness in treating anxiety or depression should not be evaluated for at least four to six weeks. As with prescription antidepressants, the effect of *Hypericum* takes place gradually. It is important to give *Hypericum* a chance. Animal studies suggest that *Hypericum* and its antidepressant effects accumulate in the brain. To discontinue treatment after one or two weeks, thinking, "This isn't working for me," is ill advised. If a satisfactory effect is not achieved in six weeks, one should consult a physician and consider taking a prescription antidepressant instead.

The National Institutes of Health's Office of Alternative Medicine, the National Institute of Mental Health, and the Office of Dietary Supplements have awarded a $4.3 million grant for a three-year study to the Department of Psychiatry at Duke University Medical Center. This will allow Duke, in the spring of 1998, to launch the first U.S. clinical trial to study *Hypericum.* The study will include 336 patients with major depression and will be coordinated by Jonathon Davidson, M.D. The patients will be randomly assigned to three treatment groups for an eight-week trial. One-third of the patients will be given a standardized 900-mg daily dose of *Hypericum;* another third will be receiving a placebo; and the last third will take Zoloft, an SSRI type of antidepressant.

Patients who respond positively will be followed for another eighteen weeks to determine which group has fewer relapses. As discussed above, Dr. Vorbach and his colleagues used 1800 mg of *Hypericum* extract daily (with no increase in side effects) for patients with major depression, twice the 900-mg daily dosage being currently considered in the Duke University study.

The neurophysiology of hunger and satiety (fullness) is complex. The hypothalamus in the brain has appetite receptors that specifically react to hunger signals conveyed by neurotransmitters. The neurotransmitter serotonin has been demonstrated to produce a feeling of fullness. High amounts of dopamine, another brain messenger, inhibit feelings of hunger. Low levels of serotonin and dopamine stimulate appetite and eating. Since *Hypericum* can enhance serotonin and dopamine activity, it may help to normalize the brain biochemistry of some people who overeat.

There is no scientific evidence, however, that *Hypericum* has any benefit as a general diet aid. For people whose binge-eating may be the result of an underlying depression or anxiety disorder, a comprehensive medical evaluation is needed before considering the use of *Hypericum*. If Saint-John's-wort is appropriate as part of a comprehensive treatment program, it must be taken in therapeutic amounts, 300 mg of extract standardized to 0.3 percent hypericin, and not the small amounts of *Hypericum* put into many diet products. *Hypericum*'s further benefits must be evaluated by medical science, rather than to treat it as a panacea.

14

Valerian—Nature's Valium—and Other Sedative Herbs

God's Valium—valerian—is a splendid sleeping pill and a fix for anxiety, and it doesn't make you feel bad later. What more could you ask?

—JEAN CARPER

As described in Part 1, anxiety makes enormous demands on the resources of both the mind and body. Accelerated heart and breath rates, increased perspiration, high levels of adrenaline and cortisol in the blood, elevated muscle tension, persistent worry, and emotional distress all take their toll on the nervous system. Chronic anxiety keeps you in a wound-up, hyperaroused state, to the point where you rarely rest well even when you finally get to sleep. As a result your mind and body have difficulty regaining their natural state of harmony, ease, and well-being. Without proper rest, the result is physical and emotional exhaustion and further vulnerability to anxiety.

Physicians have long recognized that rest plays an important role in healing. Bed rest is the usual prescription for almost all illness, from pneumonia to heart attack. The sicker you are, the more your doctor will emphatically insist that you rest. Synthetic tranquilizers and sleeping pills can provide immediate sedation but can be addictive. Also, they relieve symptoms without getting at the root of anxiety. The natural self-healing program in Part 3 will show you how to get the rest and sleep you need to heal anxiety at its core. You will learn relaxation techniques, dietary changes (including how to reduce the stimulant effects of sugar, caffeine, and cigarettes), sleep behavioral strategies, and many other ways of restoring a healthy balance of activity and rest. In addition to making these important lifestyle changes, kava, *Hypericum*, and the herbs below can help to relieve anxiety and insomnia.

VALERIAN

Valerian is as popular in herbal medicine as Valium is in pharmaceutical medicine. Yet while both are sedatives, they have nothing more in common than a similarity in spelling. Valerian is the most widely used sedative in Europe, where over one hundred valerian preparations are sold in pharmacies. Valerian is growing in popularity throughout the world because of its reputation for relieving anxiety and insomnia. Valerian (*Valeriana officinalis*) has been used for nervousness and insomnia for thousands of years in Ayurvedic medicine in India and in traditional Chinese medicine. Valerian was a very popular sleep sedative in the United States until it was displaced by synthetic drugs after World War II.

Valerian is a large perennial plant native to East India, China, Europe, and North America. The sedative substances are found in the root stock, which is dried and extracted for medicinal purposes. The safety of the valepotriates, a biochemical found in valerian, was once in question, but since these are not water soluble, they are excluded from the now standard water-soluble valerian extract. Valerian extract seems to work like benzodiazepines by enhancing the activity of gamma-aminobutyric acid (GABA), a sedative-like neurotransmitter.

Valerian has a musty, old-gym-socks aroma, but its sedative effect is nothing to wrinkle your nose at. Sound clinical and animal studies have proven valerian's capacity to induce sleep and to alleviate nightmares and abrupt awakenings. In double-blind clinical trials, valerian has reduced the amount of time it takes to fall asleep and increased the quality of sleep among a variety of patients, including poor sleepers, smokers, and habitual coffee drinkers. In double-blind, placebo-controlled studies of insomniacs, valerian has demonstrated sleep induction comparable to benzodiazepine sleeping pills but without impairing memory and concentration or causing daytime drowsiness.

A 1996 study by Gerhard and associates compared valerian to benzodiazepines and placebo in the treatment of insomnia. Side effects were reported by 50 percent of the subjects in the benzodiazepine-treated group but only 10 percent of the subjects treated with valerian. Valerian and benzodiazepines were similarly effective for alleviating insomnia.

Valerian has a long history of exceptional safety, which has been confirmed by clinical studies. In 1995 a woman in Utah attempted suicide by taking about twenty times the recommended dose. She was discharged from the hospital the next day, undamaged. While taking valerian, caution should be used when driving or operating machinery. Unlike Valiumlike drugs, valerian is not associated with dependence or addiction. While valerian is not synergistic with alcohol, it is best to be cautious in this regard. Sedatives should never be combined with alcohol. Although no cases of drug interactions have been reported, animal studies have demonstrated that valerian can potentiate the effect of phenobarbital and benzodiazepines. It can also aid in the withdrawal of benzodiazepine tranquilizers and sleeping pills, but this should only be done under a doctor's supervision.

Clinical studies on the use of valerian in insomnia have shown that valerian extract, standardized to 0.8-percent valeric acid, may be effective at a dose of 300 up to 900 mg one hour before bedtime. This herbal medicine, however, does not produce as dramatic a sedative effect as a benzodiazepine sleeping pill. The use of valerian extract can take two to three weeks before significant benefits in sleep are achieved. It may not be an appropriate medicine for acute insomnia because of this delayed onset of action. Once valerian extract takes effect, it does promote natural sleep without any risk of dependence.

Valerian extract at a dose of 50 to 100 mg taken two or three times daily has been shown to relieve performance anxiety and the stress of driving in heavy traffic. Larger doses of valerian extract may be necessary for patients who have been using benzodiazepine prescriptions for anxiety.

Germany's Commission E reports no side effects or contraindications for valerian. However, other sources report rare incidences of headaches and paradoxical stimulant-type effects, such as nervousness, restlessness, and palpitations. Valerian should not be used nightly for longer than six months.

CALMING WITH CHAMOMILE

How the doctor's brow should smile crown'd with wreaths of chamomile.

—THOMAS MOORE

Chamomile (*Matricaria recutita*) is one of the most widely used herbs in the Western world for relaxation. Chamomile has been touted for thousands of years as a calming agent and for soothing a "nervous stomach." Because of its medically proven calming effect on smooth muscle tissue, it is especially valuable when stress and anxiety cause indigestion. A 1994 study[1] showed that apigenin, an active substance in chamomile, had significant anxiolytic (antianxiety) activity. In preliminary research, apigenin was found to cause sedation by acting upon benzodiazepine (Valium-like) receptors in the brain.

Chamomile preparations are made from the flower heads, chosen just prior to blooming. Anyone with a history of allergies to ragweed, chrysanthemums, and other members of the daisy family should be careful about ingesting chamomile, but most people with ragweed allergies are not sensitive to chamomile. Hypersensitivity is rare, with less than five cases of allergic reactions to *Matricaria* reported worldwide.

Chamomile, also sometimes spelled camomile, can be found in all the ways botanicals are prepared as medicines. This herb is available in a standardized extract containing 1.2 percent apigenin and 0.5 percent essential oils. A dose of chamomile extract, taken as directed on the bottle, can serve as a mild sedative.

Chamomile tea has a long history of use as a calming drink before sleep and for menstrual cramps. However, even a strong tea, steeped in a pot for a long time, contains only about 10 percent of the sedative chemicals present in the herb. Chamomile and other herbal teas (hops, passion flower, and lemon balm) are only of use for simple relaxation or to calm a nervous stomach.

The essential oil of chamomile is frequently used in aromatherapy for stress relief. Homeopathic chamomile remedies are used for teething and colic in infants. Used externally, chamomile is found in ointments for skin inflammations (eczema, psoriasis, and sunburn) and hemorrhoids. Chamomile is as popular in Europe as ginseng is in the Orient, being found in hundreds of licensed products.

CALIFORNIA POPPY

California poppy (*Eschscholtzia californica*) is rapidly gaining popularity as a sleep aid and for easing mild anxiety. The botanical name honors Dr. Eschscholtz, a Russian physician who discovered the plant. California poppy is in the same family as the opium poppy, but it is not in the same genus. The alkaloids in California poppy are much less powerful than opiates like codeine and morphine and are not addictive. Limited clinical and pharmacological studies on California poppy confirm the plant's antianxiety and sleep-inducing properties. It is also considered to be useful for relieving nervous tension and muscle tics.

California poppy is currently sold as a tincture (a liquid extract), which can taste quite bitter, so mix it with juice. The dosage of California poppy is usually 30 drops of the tincture. Since the strengths of liquid extracts can vary, it is important to follow the manufacturer's directions on the bottle. The tea is much milder. One spoonful of the whole dried herb can be used for a cup of tea two to three times daily. California poppy and chamomile are considered safe enough for children when used as directed on the label for the appropriate age group.

HOPS

Take hops bitters three times a day, and you will have no doctor bills to pay.
—NINETEENTH-CENTURY
PATENT MEDICINE SLOGAN

The hops plant (*Humulus lupulus*) is a perennial vine that grows extensively in Germany, England, and North and South America. It bears scaly, conelike fruits, called strobiles, that have glandular hairs containing the medicinal substances. Since the eleventh century in Europe, hops have been used as a flavoring and preservative agent in the brewing of beer. They were also discovered to be a sedative when pickers were found to tire easily after accidentally ingesting them.

In modern times, a sedative chemical, dimethylvinyl carbinol, was identified in hops, accounting for the plant's reputation as a tranquilizer. Hops are best used fresh since they lose their medicinal value rapidly when stored. Like many herbs, they are very unstable when exposed to light and air. One study reported that hops lost 89 percent of their potency after nine months of storage. Hops stuffed into "dream pillows" must be fresh and changed regularly to be effective. Hops contain 0.35-percent essential oil, which is the source of the sedative chemicals. Hops is available as an extract, standardized to 5.2 percent of the alpha bitter or 2 percent of the essential oil.

Germany's Commission E has approved the use of hops flower for anxiety, restlessness, and sleep disturbances. Hops is not used for depression. Hops, particularly when combined with valerian, can promote and improve the quality of sleep. Studies show that after having taken a combination of valerian and hops at bedtime, most people have a good night's sleep and feel alert and active the following day.

PASSION FLOWER

Contrary to what is suggested by its name, passion flower (*Passiflora incarnata*), native to North America, is neither a stimulant nor an aphrodisiac but a popular herb for nervous restlessness. The name is a reference to the passion of Christ and is derived from the appearance of the flower.

In Europe, passion flower combined with valerian root is a popular remedy for insomnia, anxiety, and irritability. The calming effect of passion flower helps a person to relax and fall asleep. Research reveals no sedation the morning after. Passion flower is available in a standardized extract containing 3.5 to 4 percent isovitexin (flavonoids). 200 to 300 mg of the extract can be taken one hour before bedtime.

HERBAL MEDICINES FOR ATTENTION DEFICIT DISORDER

An estimated three and a half million children, adolescents, and adults are affected by attention deficit disorder (ADD) or attention deficit hyperactivity disorder (ADHD). Researchers have been unable to identify a specific cause, although learning disabilities, food additives (artificial coloring and preservatives), sensitivity to refined carbohydrates, nutritional deficiencies, heavy metal toxicity, and hypoglycemia have been implicated. Ritalin (methylphenidate), Dexedrine (dextroamphetamine), and synthetic antidepressants can have a 75- to 85-percent success rate but often with significant side effects. The long-term effects on a child's developing nervous system of taking these drugs have yet to be studied.

Herbal therapies, along with behavioral strategies, can serve as an alternative to pharmaceutical drugs. There is little scientific research available on the treatment of ADD/ADHD with herbs. In the absence of research, herbalists and naturopaths have developed suggestions based on traditional herbalism. The herbs most commonly used in the management of ADD/ADHD are valerian, *Hypericum*, hops, chamomile, lemon balm, ginseng, ginkgo, and lavender. These herbs are available as a tincture (a liquid extract). Mix with fresh juice as directed on the label according to the child's age. Herbal medicines as part of the overall treatment for ADD/ADHD should only be used under a doctor's supervision.

A considerable body of research exists supporting the use of dietary interventions and nutritional supplements for ADD/ADHD. Essential fatty acid (EFA) deficiencies have been documented in some cases of ADD/ADHD. There are two types of EFAs, omega-3 oils (alpha-linolenic) and omega-6 oils (cis-linoleic). All other oils that the body needs can be derived from these, but these must be present in the diet. Only primrose seed, borage seed, and black currant seed oils are high in GLA (an omega-6 derivative). Fish and flaxseed oils are high in the omega-3 oils (alpha-linolenic and eicosapentaenoic), but not GLA.

Researchers have used doses of 2 to 3 grams per day of evening primrose oil to correct the EFA deficiency noted in some ADD/ADHD children and adolescents. Although GLA content was unspecified, if the oil had nearly a 9-percent GLA content, this dosage would amount to 180 to 270 mg per day of GLA. Children and adolescents generally need more EFA supplements for correction of deficiency because of the high demand by growing bodies for EFAs. Possible stomach upset can be avoided by taking EFAs with food. No toxicity is noted for evening primrose oil or GLA.

EFAs for ADD/ADHD should certainly be considered before prescribing powerful stimulant drugs. In long-standing EFA deficiencies, treatment for three to six months may be required before therapeutic effects are seen. To learn about foods high in the various EFAs and foods that decrease the effectiveness of EFA supplements, you should consult a qualified nutritionist. For example, a nutritionist can teach you how to read food labels and avoid cottonseed oils, palm kernel, and hydrogenated fats, which can interfere with EFAs. It can also be important to avoid food dyes (especially red dye), sugar products, artificial sweeteners (such as NutraSweet), dairy products, white flour, corn, soy, fermented products using yeast, and canned or processed restaurant foods, if eating any of these is found to be associated with an ADD/ADHD child or adolescent "climbing the walls." Organically grown produce, rather than prepackaged junk foods, must become the staple of the diet.

Do not take your child off Ritalin, or any other pharmaceutical drug, without the supervision of a health professional. Again, the use of herbal medicines as part of the overall treatment for ADD/ADHD should always be done in consultation with your doctor.

15

Adaptogens— the Antistress Herbs

Adaptogens serve to recharge exhausted adrenals in today's stressed-filled world.
—DONALD J. BROWN, N.D.,
*HERBAL PRESCRIPTIONS
FOR BETTER HEALTH*

Chronic stress is a killer. It can make you vulnerable not only to anxiety but to a whole host of serious illnesses, including hypertension, heart disease, and cancer. Although you cannot avoid stress, an astounding group of herbal medicines, called *adaptogens*, can strengthen the body's ability to *adapt* to stress. Adaptogens, also called nerve tonics, help normalize the functions of the body and make it more resistant to stress.

Many people suffering from stress attempt to cope by taking tranquilizers, muscle relaxants, sleeping pills, alcohol, or recreational drugs or by smoking cigarettes. These substances can provide temporary relief, but they can soon become addicting. It is easy to develop *tolerance* to any of these drugs, which means that you need more and more of it for the same effect. These substances can temporarily numb you to the symptoms of stress, but they do not strengthen the body's stress response. On the contrary, they mostly act as depressants, further weakening the body's defenses and causing further vulnerability to stress, anxiety, and depression. The result may be addiction and toxic levels of stress.

Adaptogens protect and strengthen the body against stress from adverse situations. As defined by two Russian researchers, Drs. Brekhman and Lazarev, a substance must fulfill three criteria to qualify as an adaptogen. It must:

1. Be innocuous. It has to be harmless when used over long periods of time.
2. Increase resistance to stress; help the body cope better with any kind of adverse influence.
3. Improve performance, both physical and mental, by restoring the balance of body functions, no matter how it departs from normal.

Adaptogenic herbs contain opposing groups of constituents, each group capable of facilitating reactions in the body opposite in direction to those promoted by another group. For example, ginseng contains two fractions, Rb ginsenosides and Rg ginsenosides, which when isolated have opposite effects on blood pressure. Similarly, ginseng has another two groups of biochemical constituents, of which one can raise the blood sugar level and the other can lower it. Amazingly, the body is able to use the correct group of constituents to return to "center" and restore normal balance. In contrast, synthetic drugs are unidirectional only. Pharmaceuticals push the body in one direction to help treat an underactive or overactive disease process. For an illness, a unidirectional drug may be appropriate. To combat stress, however, an adaptogenic herb can better repair and correct the imbalance.

THE GINSENGS

Ginseng is used for repairing the five viscera, quieting the spirit, curbing the emotions, stopping agitation, removing noxious influences, brightening the eyes, enlightening the mind, and increasing wisdom. Continuous use leads one to longevity.

—TAO HUNG-CHING, 452–536 A.D.

Many of the most well-known adaptogenic herbs are subsumed under the name of ginseng: Asian ginseng (*Panax ginseng*), American ginseng (*Panax quinquefolius*), and Siberian ginseng (*Eleutherococcus senticosus*). *Panax* ginseng and Siberian ginseng have been the subject of a considerable amount of research over the last thirty years. In particular, these herbs were investigated for adaptogenic effects on the body under stress, such as physical workload, athletic performance, and exposure to chemical toxins.

Laboratory studies have shown that these herbs may improve oxygen and blood sugar metabolism as well as immune function, factors that may be of benefit in recovering from physically stressful situations. Adaptogens work best against the damaging effects of chronic stress, especially fatigue and physical exhaustion. These herbs are indicated for someone who is burned out, run down, and primarily in need of physical rejuvenation.

The ginsengs may increase the cortisol released by the adrenals during stress, an action that may not be desirable in cases of anxiety because it can stimulate the nervous system and thus increase nervousness and insomnia in susceptible individuals. Adaptogens are therefore generally not recommended during periods of acute stress and anxiety. In this regard, Siberian ginseng and American ginseng are considered milder than Asian *Panax* ginseng. The ginsengs can dramatically protect and enhance the body's ability to cope with chronic stress.

ASIAN GINSENG

Panax ginseng is one of the most popular herbal remedies in history. It is legendary for enhancing and revitalizing the healing powers of the mind and body. In continuous use for over 4000 years, it is a small perennial plant that grows in China, Japan, and Korea. Ginseng radix, the dried root and root hairs, contains the ginsenosides (also called triterpenoid saponins), the active drug constituents. High-quality wild Asian ginseng has become nearly extinct because of its popularity worldwide. A top-grade wild Asian ginseng root can cost many hundreds of dollars. *Panax ginseng* is commonly referred to as Chinese, Korean, or Asian ginseng.

Panax ginseng is the most widely used adaptogen in the world. Research has shown that Asian ginseng can protect against chronic stress and debilitating fatigue. In a placebo-controlled, double-blind study, nurses who took *Panax ginseng* when they switched from a day to a night shift demonstrated higher scores in physical and mental performance and had better moods than those on placebo. In Europe *Panax ginseng* is used in cases of diminished capacity for work and poor concentration and during convalescence from chronic illness because of its ability to aid recovery from physical stress and enhance physical performance.

Ginseng is known to increase activity in the pituitary and adrenal glands. A few studies indicate that ginseng lowers blood cholesterol and has an anticlotting action that may decrease the risk of heart attack. Ginseng is not used as a cure for specific diseases but has a long-standing reputation as an antiaging and antisenility remedy. Especially in elderly patients, research has confirmed that ginseng can improve vitality, alertness, concentration, coordination, memory, and mood. Its apparent cardiotonic, cancer-prevention, immune-stimulating, and liver-protecting benefits might lend credence to claims that ginseng can promote longevity.

Commission E does not report any contraindications for ginseng root. It is generally safe when used in moderation and as directed. This herb is not appropriate for everyone, however. Anyone with an anxiety disorder, manic-depressive illness, heart palpitations, asthma, or emphysema should not take Asian ginseng. Also, expectant mothers should not take ginseng. The use of ginseng in combination with other stimulants, such as caffeine or ephedra, is discouraged for people with high blood pressure or migraine headaches and in acute phases of illness. Side effects are uncommon but, if high doses of *Panax ginseng* are taken, can include insomnia, heart palpitations, high blood pressure, gastrointestinal upset, and diarrhea. In female users there are also rare cases of breast pain, possible postmenopausal bleeding, and changes in menstrual cycling.

The usual dosage, based on research studies, is 100 mg of ginseng extract standardized to 13 percent ginsenosides twice daily. If ginseng powder is used, research cites a dosage of 1500 mg per day in divided doses. Many researchers suggest a two weeks on, two weeks off dose schedule.

AMERICAN GINSENG

American ginseng is especially appropriate for American people because it can help counteract stress while supporting the adrenal system and strengthening digestion. This can lead to higher energy levels. Americans today with their fast-paced lifestyles are sadly in need of such support.

—CHRISTOPHER HOBBS, *THE GINSENGS*

Panax quinquefolius is traditionally considered somewhat milder and less stimulating than Asian ginseng. Native Americans traditionally used it as a strengthener of mental powers as well as a remedy for nausea and vomiting. Daniel Boone helped export American ginseng, and the Astor family began making its fortune by shipping it to China.

The native American species of ginseng has been so sought after in the wild that it has been declared an endangered species. Its collection and sale require a permit. As a result, wild American ginseng is very expensive. The price is driven not only by its scarcity but by the demand for it in urban Asia as they have found their own ginseng too stimulating for sedentary urban lifestyles. The cultivated variety is much less costly but requires as long as five years to produce a mature root. Cultivated American ginseng, exported from the United States (primarily from Wisconsin) and Canada (primarily from British Columbia), has become highly esteemed by Asians.

Compared to Asian ginseng, American ginseng is considered "cooler," or less stimulating, by herbalists and therefore thought to be more appropriate for counteracting the stress experienced by overworked, burned-out, adrenally depleted young adults. Asian ginseng is considered "warmer," or more stimulating, and therefore thought better suited for those over fifty. American ginseng is often touted as "cool," but this is incorrect. It is "cooler" than Asian ginseng but still stimulating.

Because of the lack of specific research on American ginseng, most herbalists default to the studies of Asian ginseng for safety guidelines. People with acute anxiety or asthma should not take American or Asian ginseng. The usual dosage is 100 mg of ginseng extract standardized to 13 percent ginsenosides two times daily. A two weeks on, two weeks off schedule is recommended.

SIBERIAN GINSENG (ELEUTHERO)

Extensively researched over the last thirty years, and with a 2000-year-old history of use, Siberian ginseng is emerging as one of the best documented "new" medicinal plants of the late twentieth century.

—STEVEN FOSTER, *HERBS FOR YOUR HEALTH*

While Siberian ginseng (*Eleutherococcus senticosus*, also called eleuthero) is a model adaptogen, it is not a species of *Panax* and is therefore not a traditional ginseng. The active constituents, called eleutherosides, are located in the root and have many of the same tonic effects as *Panax* ginseng. Beginning in the 1950s, Russian research popularized eleuthero as a relatively low-cost substitute for *Panax* ginseng. Soviet cosmonauts and Olympic athletes reportedly used it to boost endurance, performance, and stamina.

Siberian ginseng appears to have a broad spectrum of benefits, which include promoting adaptation to climactic extremes of heat, cold, and altitude, increasing workload, improving visual and aural acuity, and protecting against radiation and decompression. It restores homeostasis to stressed adrenal and pituitary glands.

Eleuthero appears to strongly enhance the immune system. A 1977 study was done on 1000 citizens of the former Soviet Union who held stressful jobs, such as merchant sailors, deep sea divers, telegraph operators, rescue workers, airplane pilots, and proofreaders. They took Siberian ginseng extract for five separate one-month periods and showed increased stamina, endurance, and general health, as measured by about a 40-percent reduction in lost work days and a 50-percent reduction in general illness.

Eleuthero is better suited than *Panax* ginseng for people suffering from mild anxiety and insomnia. Studies of patients with symptoms of neurosis (such as a general state of anxiety), irritability, and extreme exhaustion showed a significant increase in well-being following treatment with eleuthero extract. German health authorities allow Siberian ginseng to be labeled as an invigorating tonic against stress and for fortification in times of fatigue, debility, and convalescence. Other approved uses are for decreased work capacity and diminished concentration.

The only listed contraindication for eleuthero is high blood pressure, but significant research in this area is absent. There are no significant side effects or interactions with other drugs. Eleuthero, like *Panax* ginseng, can be stimulating, so don't take it too close to bedtime. As is true for all ginsengs, if it should make you tense or anxious, reduce your dosage or stop taking the herb.

Much of the Russian research on Siberian ginseng used one to three doses of 0.5 to 6.0 ml of a 33-percent alcohol extract, now widely available in the United States. For stamina and performance benefits, 2 to 8 ml per day in divided doses are recommended. The extract of Siberian ginseng is standardized to contain 0.3 percent of eleutheroside B and 0.5 percent of eleutheroside E, for a total of 0.8 percent eleutherosides. The usual dose of the extract is 180 to 360 mg a day in divided doses for a period of two to three months, followed by a two-week break. Harmonex, a new supplement from Sunsource, combines Siberian ginseng extract and Saint-John's-wort extract to help maintain physical and emotional balance.

MILK THISTLE

This herbal adaptogen is widely used in European medicine to enhance the liver's adaptation to the toxic stresses of modern life. Some of the synthetic antidepressants and other prescription drugs used to treat anxiety can damage the liver. Even moderate alcohol consumption can injure this vital organ, necessary for detoxifying harmful chemicals. The liver serves to protect your internal environment.

In over two hundred medical studies, milk thistle (*Silybum marianum*) has been shown to prevent and reverse the liver damage caused by environmental pollutants, chemical pesticides, automobile exhaust, and other toxic by-products of the industrialized era. Recent studies published in the *Journal of the American Medical Association (JAMA)* have shown that 78 percent of adult Americans have sub-clinical evidence of chronic liver damage. Even a slight amount of liver impairment can cause irritability, malaise, fatigue, and subtle mental impairment. Indeed, some researchers consider the massive amounts of environmental poisons to be a major contributor to the modern epidemics of anxiety and depression.

Almost 2000 years ago, the Greek physician Dioscorides and the Roman naturalist Pliny recommended milk thistle to treat liver disorders from toxic poisoning. Used as a medicine since ancient times, this thistle-topped weed, with a prickly purplish flower, contains large amounts of flavonoids, extraordinarily therapeutic biochemicals. Silymarin, a group of the most potent flavonoids, was isolated in 1968 from the seeds and the fruits of the flower. This powerful antioxidant continues to astound the medical world. Extensive research has demonstrated that silymarin can protect liver cells from harmful free radicals (see page 50) and toxic chemicals, and stimulate their regeneration when they are damaged.

Medical studies have substantiated milk thistle's value for treating both acute and chronic liver disorders, such as hepatitis, cirrhosis, and toxicity from carbon tetrachloride, high-dose Tylenol (acetaminophen), iron overload, and the deadly poison of the amanita mushroom. This herb can be especially therapeutic for a liver damaged by alcohol. Milk thistle can lower abnormally elevated liver enzymes, the laboratory marker of alcohol-damaged liver cells, by as much as 80 percent. Of course, for milk thistle to be most effective, abstinence from alcohol is also necessary.

Healing anxiety sometimes means recovering from some of the synthetic drugs that have been used to treat it. For those taking pharmaceutical antianxiety drugs, such as phenothiazines, butyrophenones, and certain antidepressants, milk thistle can help counter some of the damage these may cause the liver. Indeed, you should discuss with your doctor taking milk thistle to help offset the side effects of any prescribed drug that can potentially harm the liver, such as the cholesterol-reducing drugs Zocor (simvastatin) and Mevacor (lovastatin).

The best milk thistle to take is a guaranteed potency extract standardized to contain 80-percent silymarin. A 200-mg pill of milk thistle extract standardized to provide 80-percent silymarin contains 160 mg of silymarin. The most commonly used dosage is 160 mg of silymarin three times daily. If your liver has signs of damage, you should take milk thistle extract only under the supervision of your physician. After you show improvement, as documented by liver function blood tests, silymarin extract can be cut down to 160 mg twice a day. In cases of liver damage from alcohol, it can take two months of milk thistle extract treatment, plus abstinence, before elevated liver enzymes are lowered. For chronic liver problems, Germany's Commission E recommends taking 160 mg of silymarin extract daily. Taking 320 mg of silymarin extract daily in two divided doses is recommended by some European doctors for people who have a higher risk of liver toxicity, such as those who drink more alcohol than they should or who work around industrial chemicals.

In therapeutic doses, the use of milk thistle extract is remarkably well tolerated, even in patients with serious liver disease. Medical studies have shown that it causes only mild side effects, such as gastrointestinal discomfort and loose stools, in less than 1 percent of users. Milk thistle even in large doses appears to be nontoxic. It produces no allergic reactions and does not interact with other medications. Commission E does not warn against the use of milk thistle during pregnancy and lactation. While milk thistle can strengthen the liver's adaptation to the pollutants and poisons of modern life, we must also curb alcohol abuse and the causes of a toxic environment.

16

Ginkgo biloba—
Antidote to
the Angst of Aging

> *The goal of life is to die young—as late as possible.*
>
> —ASHLEY MONTAGU, PH.D.

The baby-boomer generation was somehow programmed to never grow old. Raised with unrealistic expectations of life after fifty, millions of members of this generation are now suffering from the angst of aging. With a life expectancy of seventy-five, fears of mental deterioration loom large. As a result, there is enormous interest in the emerging science of enhancing and protecting the aging brain.

"Paying attention to the brain and its needs makes a difference," say John Ratey, M.D., and Catherine Johnson, Ph.D., of Harvard University Medical School. "If we are successful, we may become the first generation of centenarians who not only know exactly where we put the car keys but still have a license—and a reason—to drive." Studies have shown that what go first in normal aging are the sense of direction and spatial relations, cognitive skills that are necessary to find your car in a supermall parking lot. The potential for still remembering where we parked at the age of one hundred is an exciting prospect for those with "anxious aging," including the worry about worrying about these things!

There is perhaps no greater threat to the hope of aging gracefully than Alzheimer's disease. The fear of developing this illness has been heightened by watching the decline of former President Ronald Reagan. The desire to avoid becoming a part of this growing epidemic, as well as the general angst of aging, has made almost everyone interested in preventing Alzheimer's. To help the brain keep fit, Americans are taking an array of memory potions and elixirs of youth. New research suggests that one of them, the best-studied and popular herb, *Ginkgo biloba,* can truly make a difference. Ginkgo sales topped $163 million in Germany in 1996 and are rapidly reaching the same level in America.

Ginkgo biloba extract could be an invaluable aid in the treatment and prevention of Alzheimer's disease.
—DANIEL B. MOWREY, PH.D.

Ginkgo is the oldest living tree species in the world, having survived unchanged in China for over three hundred million years. Charles Darwin called the gingko tree a living fossil. Ginkgo trees, also known as maidenhair trees, are very resistant to viruses, fungi, insects, pollution, and even radiation. In fact, a ginkgo tree was the only plant to survive the atomic bomb dropped on Hiroshima. The great longevity of the ginkgo has made it a popular ornamental tree in parks and along the streets of U.S. cities. Individual trees can live for more than a thousand years. Just as this hardy tree can live to a ripe old age, *Ginkgo biloba* extract can help a generation of baby boomers to overcome their angst and die young—as late as possible.

The October 22, 1997 *Journal of the American Medical Association* published research which showed that *Ginkgo biloba* extract appears to slow Alzheimer's disease. The randomly assigned, double-blind, placebo-controlled study was performed for one year by neurologist Dr. Pierre L. LeBars and a team of scientists at the New York Institute for Medical Research. The researchers found that 27 percent of patients who took 120 mg of ginkgo extract for six months or longer improved their mental functioning, including memory, reasoning, and the ability to learn, compared to only 14 percent of those taking placebo. The study began with 309 patients aged 45 or older with most suffering from Alzheimer's disease but also some with dementia caused by strokes. Ginkgo is by no means a miracle cure for Alzheimer's. The study showed that ginkgo can stabilize or even improve mental performance in one-third of those who are mildly impaired by Alzheimer's.

The particular form of *Ginkgo biloba* extract used in the study is called Egb761, and it is widely used in Europe for the treatment of Alzheimer's. German studies have demonstrated that 240 mg of Egb761 a day is perhaps more effective than the 120 mg daily dose used in the *JAMA* study for the treatment of Alzheimer's. The most potent ginkgo formulations use a strictly controlled process developed in Germany. The Egb761 used in this study was supplied by the Murdock-Madaus-Schwabe Company in Springville, Utah. The extract is sold in the United States under the trade names Ginkgold and Ginkgo-D.

NATURAL BRAIN BOOSTER

Ginkgo increases blood flow to the brain and has excellent restorative effects on the nervous system. Hundreds of scientific studies, involving tens of thousands of patients, attest to the effectiveness of *Ginkgo biloba* extract for the many problems associated with cerebral vascular insufficiency and impaired mental performance in elderly patients. The active components of *Ginkgo biloba* have a profound tonic effect on the mind and body. Egb761 has been shown to inhibit the reuptake of norepinephrine, serotonin, dopamine, and acetylcholine, important neurotransmitters in the brain. The extract acts as an antioxidant and a nerve cell membrane stabilizer. It also enhances oxygen and glucose utilization and increases blood flow in arteries, veins, and capillaries. Experiments involving learned helplessness and behavioral despair in laboratory animals demonstrated that Egb761 exhibited some antianxiety and antidepressant activities. Ginkgo is of benefit for many of the presumed symptoms of aging:

- Anxiety and depression
- Memory impairment
- Poor concentration, decreased alertness
- Diminished intellectual capacity
- Vertigo, headache
- Tinnitus (ringing in the ears)
- Macular degeneration (the most common cause of blindness in adults)
- Inner ear disturbances (which can cause partial deafness)
- Poor circulation in the extremities
- Impotence due to impaired penile blood flow

A concentrated extract is needed because large doses of the herb are required for the medicinal effects. It is standardized to 24-percent ginkgo flavone glycosides. Unless otherwise prescribed, take one 60-mg tablet two times a day with water. It has to be taken consistently for at least six weeks to be effective, but the longer ginkgo extract is used, the greater the benefit.

Ginkgo extract is considered relatively safe and remarkably free of side effects when taken as directed. Some people who take extremely large doses may have diarrhea, nausea, vomiting, dizziness, and restlessness. If this should occur, reduce the dosage. If side effects are severe, discontinue it. *Ginkgo biloba* extract acts as a blood thinner by inhibiting platelets from clumping together, so it could be unsafe for patients who are taking aspirin or other blood thinners. In Europe, ginkgo extract is prescribed in lower doses (40 mg daily) for patients who are taking aspirin or anticoagulants for circulatory problems.

In addition to the 1997 report in the *Journal of the American Medical Association*, other studies on ginkgo have appeared in such diverse journals as *Lancet, Audiology*, and the *Journal of Urology*. Over 120,000 physicians worldwide write over ten million prescriptions for ginkgo each year, accounting for over five hundred million dollars in sales. In addition to the uses listed above, European doctors prescribe it as part of the treatments for premenstrual syndrome, attention deficit disorder, multiple sclerosis, diabetic tissue damage, Raynaud's phenomenon, and intermittent claudication. Ginkgo is not specifically recommended as a treatment for anxiety and depression, except when they may be symptoms secondary to aging or cerebrovascular insufficiency.

17

Herbs in Traditional Chinese Medicine

> *The differences between traditional Chinese and Western medicine have to do with the ways in which diseases are perceived, diagnosed, and treated. It remains to be seen how the two systems compare in terms of efficacy. But the systems need not be mutually exclusive. There is no reason why physicians cannot combine the finest elements of both schools. A Chinese proverb says, "The methods used by one man may be faulty. The methods used by two men will be better."*
>
> —DAVID EISENBERG, M.D.

Ancient Chinese medicine prescribed *Ginkgo biloba* to rejuvenate the brain nearly 5,000 years ago. Traditional Chinese medicine (TCM) is one of the oldest written medical systems that has codified the use of herbs. In 2800 B.C., the Emperor Shen Nong, a Chinese herbalist, recorded the *Pen Ts'ao Ching*, a list of hundreds of medicinal plants, which included ginkgo, creating the oldest known Chinese pharmacopoeia. Currently TCM is worth trying for a wide range of chronic disorders, including anxiety that has been resistant to other types of treatment.

Chinese herbalism is based upon a dualistic Taoist philosophy. Yin and yang are the two opposing forces present in all of creation, including people and herbs. Yang is warm, bright, dominant, and masculine, while yin is cool, dim, yielding, and feminine. Every human being has to maintain a balance of yin and yang to enjoy good health and harmony. Excessive stress and anxiety can result in yin deficiency. To restore the balanced interaction of yin and yang, TCM uses not only herbs but also massage, dietary change, *qigong* exercises, and acupuncture. Acupuncture is used to treat a wide range of conditions including anxiety and stress. The treatment apparently stimulates the production of endorphins, opiate-like substances in the brain.

An interesting social phenomenon is the growing popularity of "elixir bars," serving herbal tonics to consumers. These plush, pleasant bars offer their customers the Eastern equivalent of coffee-on-the-run. Establishments such as the Three Treasures Elixir Bar in Beverly Hills, the Gan Bei Tonic Bar in West Hollywood and the Dragon's Light in Denver provide a variety of elixir drinks made from TCM herbal extracts.

Traditional Chinese herbs, such as *Panax ginseng*, *Ginkgo biloba*, and licorice root (see below), are primarily taken to promote health rather than to treat a specific disease. The Chinese pharmacopoeia has a vast number of herbs that are frequently combined in a synergistic balance to enhance benefits. Many Chinese herbs that appear to have significant medicinal value are being scrutinized by Western pharmacologists. Modern scientific inquiry into TCM is already yielding more plant medicines for stress and anxiety, including the herbs below.

REISHI FOR RELAXATION — A MEDICINAL MUSHROOM

Traditionally, reishi was used in China by Taoist monks to promote a centered calmness, improve meditative practices, and attain a long and healthy life.

—ROY UPTON, FOUNDER,
AMERICAN HERBAL
PHARMACOPOEIA FOUNDATION

Reishi (*Ganoderma lucidum*), one of the most famous medicinal mushrooms of ancient China, has recently become popular in the United States for reducing anxiety and insomnia. *Lucidum* refers to the bright, shiny surface of the fungus's fruiting body. Reishi is known as *ling-zhi* in China, which means "spirit plant." The Chinese and Japanese have used reishi since ancient times to treat various medical problems, including high blood pressure, neurasthenia, bronchitis, asthma, and liver disease. Recent studies have found that among the active substances in reishi are triterpene acids, which decrease hypertension, and polysaccharides, which have antibacterial and anti-inflammatory effects.

Reishi mushrooms and prescription antihypertensive drugs can be an effective combination, according to recent research at universities in China and Japan. Double-blind, placebo-controlled studies showed that when a reishi extract was given along with antihypertensive drugs, there was a significant decrease in blood pressure. Reishi may be a particularly suitable relaxant for people with high blood pressure, but more research is needed.

Herbalist Christopher Hobbs in his book *Medicinal Mushrooms* (Botanica Press, 1995) states that reishi "is especially suitable as a calming herb for people with anxiety, sleeplessness or nervousness accompanied by adrenal weakness." He cautions that hemophiliacs should avoid using reishi because of its high adenosine content.

Reishi extract is standardized to 4 percent triterpenes and 10 percent polysaccharides. Dosage of reishi extract should be discussed with your doctor. The usual dose is a 250 to 350 mg tablet of mushroom extract three times daily. Do not take reishi for longer than two to three months, because there are few studies on its long-term effects. At the start of treatment with reishi, side effects can include achiness, increased bowel movements (which usually subside within days), vertigo, and eruptions or itchiness of the skin. Reishi interacts with the sedative drugs chlorpromazine (Thorazine) and barbiturates.

Another TCM mushroom is cordyceps, known in China as the caterpillar fungus. This mushroom is a nontoxic herbal tonic that is particularly useful for people coping with excessive stress. Dried cordyceps can be taken as an extract or tea to increase energy and stamina; just follow the directions on the label. Also, Chinese green tea, used as a meditative aid in twelfth-century Zen monasteries, is a marvelous calming tea.

LICORICE ROOT FOR CHRONIC FATIGUE SYNDROME

The stress of daily living can naturally make you tired and sometimes exhausted. Chronic fatigue syndrome (CFS), however, is characterized by chronic intense fatigue. It sometimes begins with a perplexing flulike illness. The person soon becomes bedridden with debilitating fatigue, accompanied by symptoms such as enlarged, painful lymph nodes, headaches, joint and muscle aches, anxiety, and difficulty concentrating. Hundreds of thousands of Americans suffer from CFS, whose cause is still unknown. Rather than attempt to self-diagnose, you should always consult your doctor.

In 1995 Dr. Hugh Calkins and his colleagues at the Johns Hopkins Medical School discovered that CFS is sometimes associated with neurally mediated hypotension, a type of low blood pressure abnormality. This disorder causes the blood pressure to drop swiftly when a person stands, causing light-headedness and sometimes fainting. In the study, 22 out of the 23 CFS patients had this condition. Neurally mediated hypotension can be definitively diagnosed with a tilt-table test, used to suspend the patient in an upright position while blood pressure is monitored.

Health writer Jean Carper, in her book *Miracle Cures* (HarperCollins, 1997), reported that licorice root can relieve the symptoms of some CFS patients with neurally mediated hypotension. Licorice (*Glycyrrhiza glabra*) has been used in TCM for over 5000 years, as recorded in the *Pen Ts'ao Ching*. TCM practitioners consider licorice root to be a key herb for health and use it in their herbal combinations perhaps even more than ginseng. Renowned herbal scholar Daniel B. Mowrey, Ph.D., called licorice "one of the two or three most important herbs in the world."

Licorice root as a medicine must be the genuine article. The licorice candy in America is actually made from anise and typically contains no real licorice root. Glycyrrhizic acid, an important active component of licorice root, is a natural corticosteroid, with activity closely resembling cortisone. Like steroids, licorice root can raise blood pressure. It is this property that makes licorice a valuable treatment for CFS patients with neurally mediated hypotension. The tilt-table test can be valuable to find the exact dose of licorice root that normalizes blood pressure. The use of licorice root to treat this condition, or any other medical disorder, should be monitored by a physician.

According to a 1991 study by Dr. Mark Demitrack and his colleagues at the University of Michigan Medical Center, about two-thirds of CFS patients have mild adrenal insufficiency, as shown by significantly reduced basal evening glucocorticoid levels, low 24-hour urinary free cortisol excretion, and elevated adrenocorticotropic hormone (ACTH). Adrenal insufficiency could not only cause neurally mediated hypotension but also account for the classic symptoms of CFS, such as slowly progressive fatigue, asthenia (weakness), suppressed immune response, joint and muscle aches, and difficulty concentrating.

The adrenal insufficiency of CFS is usually treated with synthetic steroids like Florinef (fludrocortisone). Licorice root has also been used effectively to treat this condition and may be safer. Since treatment of adrenal insufficiency may require large amounts of cortisone, an attractive alternative might be the addition of licorice root to reduce the required dosage of synthetic steroids.

Licorice root is not appropriate for everyone with CFS, however. People with hypertension should not take licorice, because it could further raise their blood pressure, perhaps dangerously. Even people with normal blood pressure who ingest inappropriately large amounts of licorice root can develop serious hypertension. Licorice should not be taken by anyone with heart disease, diabetes, glaucoma, or depression. Because licorice can raise blood cortisol, it can worsen a depression, a condition that can easily be mistaken for CFS. Licorice should not be used unless you have enlarged, painful lymph nodes and laboratory tests show that you have low blood cortisol levels (adrenal insufficiency).

People being treated with licorice extract should be monitored for low potassium, which if unrecognized can lead to sudden cardiac arrest.

Caution: Some imported European licorice candies contain potent extracts of the plant. An overdose of licorice, though rare, can cause heart failure, requiring urgent medical attention.

Licorice is available in health food stores in capsules or liquid extracts standardized for glycyrrhizic acid content. It should only be taken by CFS patients in consultation with a doctor. When licorice is taken appropriately, the Food and Drug Administration considers its long-term use to be generally safe. If your physician recommends that you take licorice extract for CFS, be sure not to use deglycyrrhizinated licorice (DGL). Licorice with the glycyrrhizin molecule removed is no longer effective for CFS. After adrenal insufficiency in CFS patients is corrected with licorice extract, the herbal adaptogens Asian and Siberian ginseng can be used for long-term support of normal pituitary and adrenal gland functioning.

18

Herbs in Ayurvedic Medicine

You Herbs, born at the birth of time,
More ancient than the gods themselves,
O Plants, with this hymn I sing to you,
Our mothers and our gods.

—RIG VEDA

Ayurveda comes from the Sanskrit meaning "science of life" and is the world's oldest continually practiced system of medicine, dating back over 5000 years in India. The *Veda*, which literally means "knowledge" or "science," makes numerous references to the use of herbs for healing and rejuvenation. Ayurvedic medicine practitioners routinely prescribe herbs as a part of treatment. Ayurvedic herbs are matched not only to a specific illness but to your *dosha*, or characteristic metabolic (mind-body) type. The three doshas are *vata*, responsible for all movement in the body, *pitta*, responsible for metabolism, and *kapha*, responsible for bodily structure.

According to this system, when your *vata* becomes imbalanced, you are particularly prone to anxiety, worry, insomnia, generalized aches and pains, and depression. *Vata* imbalances account for the enormous number of prescriptions written in the Western world for tranquilizers, sleeping pills, and pain relievers. Indeed, *vata* aggravation is considered to be the most common disorder in America. Many Ayurvedic practitioners compound custom herbal formulas, tailored from well-known classic formulas, to help bring *vata* into balance. Ashwaganda, Shanka puspi (*Convolvulus mycrophyllus*), and Brahmi (*Hydrocetyle asiatica*) are popular Ayurvedic herbs to relieve anxiety. Some ayurvedic products contain a lot of sugar, which may pose a problem for some patients with hypoglycemia or diabetes.

The goal of Ayurveda is not just to eliminate symptoms but to balance the *dosha* and integrate body, mind, and spirit. Meditation, yoga, diet, exercise, soothing music, massage, and lifestyle changes to eliminate alcohol, caffeine, and nicotine are also considered essential to balancing *vata*. Ayurvedic medicine also uses aromas, such as rose, geranium, and orange essential oils, to balance *vata*. *Pranayama*, Ayurvedic respiratory exercises, are used to restore balance to the breathing of anxious individuals. *Abhyangas* are self-administered daily massages with oil to reduce nervousness and restore harmony. *Panchakarma* uses herbal oil preparations in special massages to cleanse, detoxify, and rejuvenate. Part of the *panchakarma* purification program offered at an Ayurvedic health center is *shirodhara*, warm sesame oil slowly poured onto your forehead and then used for a head massage. This treatment can be a highly pleasurable form of anxiety relief.

Maharishi Mahesh Yogi, founder of the Transcendental Meditation program, revived Ayurveda and brought it to the West in 1985, as Maharishi Ayur-Veda. Deepak Chopra, M.D., developed his own program of Ayurvedic healing in 1990. Ayurvedic herbs and natural treatment programs are available from Maharishi Ayur-Veda and the Chopra Center for Well Being (see appendix C).

ASHWAGANDA

*Ayurvedic medicine incorporates many herbs and tech-
niques for reducing stress. One of the foremost herbs
used for stress is Ashwaganda, which is highly reputed
as an effective nervine sedative and anxiolytic (anxiety
reducer).*
                                    —SCOTT GERSON, M.D.

Ashwaganda (*Withania somnifera*) is an Ayurvedic herb
known for its rejuvenating powers and for calming anxiety. It
can reduce stress and enhance vitality, learning, and memory.
A 1997 clinical study demonstrated that ashwaganda reduced
the level of plasma cortisol and was beneficial for patients
with anxiety neurosis. A 1993 clinical study showed that ashwaganda improved mood and increased hemoglobin and
blood plasma protein levels. Another study in 1995 showed
that ashwaganda could help to alleviate the severe stress of
morphine withdrawal.

There is also research on immune system benefits of ashwaganda. This may be particularly important in light of the
fact that stress is often associated with immunosuppression.
Ashwaganda is frequently and mistakenly referred to as Indian
ginseng because of its ability to strengthen and tone the nervous system.

Ashwaganda extract standardized to contain 1.5 percent
withanolides and 1 percent alkaloids should be taken as
directed on the bottle. It can cause some mild gastrointestinal complaints, which can usually be alleviated by taking
the herb with meals. Ashwaganda should not be taken with
barbiturates. For stress protection, ashwaganda is often
blended with two other popular Indian herbs, *Gotu kola* and
Shatavari (Indian asparagus), and also with Siberian ginseng.

Hygienics, purity, and standardization are legitimate concerns because herbal products from India have a reputation for contamination with animal feces, insects, and mold. Ashwaganda extract is now being supplied by Nature's Way, TwinLab, and other reputable American companies that enforce strict sanitation standards.

AN ANCIENT
ANTIPSYCHOTIC HERB

Over two millennia before chlorpromazine was synthesized, ancient India was already using an herbal antipsychotic: Rauvolfia serpentina.
—VINOD S. BHATARA; J.N. SHARMA;
SANJAY GUPTA; AND Y.K. GUPTA,
AMERICAN JOURNAL OF PSYCHIATRY, JULY 1997

Folk medicinal use of serpentwood (*Rauvolfia serpentina*) led to the discovery of reserpine, the first known antipsychotic. The potency of this herb makes it inappropriate for self-medication today. It was prescribed for abnormal mental conditions in India over 2000 years ago, as described in ancient Ayurvedic medical texts. The dried roots, known as the insanity herb, were used as a treatment for a wide variety of mental disorders.

In 1937 Drs. Sen, Bose, and Gupta reported that *Rauvolfia serpentina* was a powerful tranquilizer. In 1953 Dr. Hakim, from Ahrnabad, India, was awarded a gold medal for his paper detailing a cure of schizophrenia with *Rauvolfia serpentina*. In 1952 reserpine was isolated from *Rauvolfia serpentina* and found to have a remarkably calming effect on humans and animals. Today reserpine is no longer an appropriate treatment for psychosis, owing to side effects, a long delay in action, a tendency to induce or intensify depression, and the availability of much better medicines.

Yet reserpine and its analogues are still used today in the management of mild to moderate hypertension. Germany's Commission E approves *Rauvolfia serpentina* for mild essential high blood pressure, especially when associated with anxiety. However, it has numerous side effects, interacts negatively with various drugs, and is contraindicated for depression, ulcers, pregnancy, and lactation. In the treatment of hypertension, there are much better options. *Rauvolfia serpentina*'s remarkable history does illustrate, however, the importance of continuing to research Ayurvedic herbs. Although these herbs remain little known outside India, and just a few have been scientifically investigated, many appear to have significant therapeutic value.

19

Herbal Scents—
Aromatherapy

> *I should like to raise the question whether*
> *the inevitable stunting of the sense of smell*
> *as a result of man's turning away from the*
> *earth, and the organic repression of the*
> *smell-pleasure produced by it, does not*
> *largely share in his predisposition to ner-*
> *vous diseases.*
>
> —SIGMUND FREUD

Smells act directly on the brain, like drugs. Every breath you take passes currents of air molecules over the nerve receptors in your nose. Five million cells in your nasal cavities fire impulses directly to the olfactory area of your brain and from there to the hypothalamus and limbic system, the seat of your emotions. The sense of smell is so powerfully connected to the brain that some scents can elicit pronounced changes in an area of the brain called the hippocampus, responsible for memory. This is why an odor can sometimes bring back past memories so vividly. Pleasant fragrances prompt us to take slower, deeper breaths and become measurably more relaxed. Which natural scents do you find calming and relaxing? Which elicit peaceful or happy memories?

The amygdala, the alarm center located in the limbic system, can be strongly influenced by specific scents. Lavender can help promote deeper, more restful sleep, apparently by activating the neurotransmitter serotonin. You might set a small bowl of potpourri naturally scented with lavender or rose petals on your nightstand for a more restful sleep. Research at Rensselaer Polytechnic Institute in Troy, New York, indicates that people who work in pleasantly scented areas show a 25 percent increase in performance over those not exposed. They carry out tasks more confidently, more efficiently, and with fewer errors. Freshly cut flowers or a naturally scented herbal potpourri can refresh and renew you at home or work.

Aromatherapy is a system of healing the body with aromatic essences of plant extracts called essential oils. These oils turn from a liquid to a gas very easily at room temperature or when warmed. Essential oils have been used to maintain health and alleviate tension for thousands of years, going back to ancient Egypt and China.

The term *aromatherapy* was coined in 1937 by René-Maurice Gattefossé, a French chemist, who revived the tradition of aromatic treatments. Controlled brain-wave studies by researchers at Toho University in Japan have yielded remarkable data about how specific scents tend to stimulate or relax. Smelling jasmine keeps people more alert and improves performance, correlating with increased beta waves in the frontal cortex. The scent of lavender, on the other hand, which induces relaxation, is associated with increased alpha waves in the back of the head.

Aromatherapy, particularly the use of lavender oil to relax patients, is practiced widely at Churchill Hospital in Oxford, England. Nurses there use lavender oil, vaporized or applied by massage, to help reduce anxiety and induce sleep without sedatives, according to the *International Journal of Aromatherapy*. A recent study in *Lancet*, a prestigious British medical journal, reported that insomniacs slept through the night when their bedrooms were scented with lavender.

The mood-altering power of essential oils can be of therapeutic benefit for anxiety, insomnia, and nervous tension. Soothing essential oils, such as lavender, chamomile, neroli, bergamot, sweet marjoram, and ylang-ylang, can be used alone or in combination for stress relief and to help calm hyperactive children.

Using essential oils can be as simple as smelling the oils from the bottle or applying a few drops to the hands or wrists. Be careful about applying undiluted essential oils to the skin, however, because they are extremely concentrated and may cause irritation. For best results, make a 10-percent dilution of 10 drops of essential oil in an ounce of carrier oil such as sweet almond, olive, safflower, or sesame seed. For a longer lasting scent you can use a small scent dispenser, an aroma lamp, or an electric aromatherapy essential oil room diffuser.

To achieve the desired results in aromatherapy, be sure to buy your essential oils from a manufacturer that specializes in pure plant essential oils. Many essential oils on the market are adulterated or stretched with less expensive or synthetic oils. Perfume or fragrance oils are almost always synthetics and will not produce therapeutic benefits. Cosmetic companies such as the Body Shop, Esteé Lauder, and Origins carry synthetic fragrance oils, which are not recommended for aromatherapy.

HERBAL BATHS AND MASSAGE OILS

The way to health is to have an aromatic bath and a scented massage every day.

—HIPPOCRATES

A hot herbal bath can be a wonderful antidote to a hectic, high-pressured pace. Enjoy an herbal bath instead of a shower, especially when you are stressed. Essential oils are highly concentrated and potent herbal substances. It takes about a hundred pounds of plant matter to extract an ounce of oil. Pure rose oil, made from hundreds of pounds of petals, is very expensive. Natural vanilla is also costly. Lavender, ylang-ylang, neroli, geranium, and patchouli are less expensive and can be just as effective for a relaxing herbal bath.

Herbal baths should be approached in an unhurried and meditative state. Draw a warm bath (about 100 degrees) to neck level, and put in 2 to 15 drops, depending on the oil. Use more of a milder oil, such as lavender, but less of a potentially irritating oil, such as peppermint. For even deeper cleansing and to maintain the skin's acid mantle, add ½ cup of unprocessed apple cider vinegar to the bath.

Essential oils can be massaged into the skin. Remember to use a 10-percent dilution, as described above. It is possible to have an allergic reaction to essential oils. Spice oils such as thyme, sage, and oregano can be particularly irritating, while floral oils are generally mild. Be sure not to get essential oils in the eyes when applying the massage mixture, because they can be irritating. If this should happen, soak a cotton swab with vegetable oil, hold it in the corner of the eye, and carefully wipe the lids. Also, do not take essential oils internally. If pregnant, avoid all essential oils in the first trimester. After that, stick to gentle floral oils such as lavender, rose, and chamomile.

20

Flower Power

The Bach flower remedies are a system of natural medicine developed in the 1930s that uses thirty-eight flowering plants and trees, prepared with a specific homeopathic process, to treat and prevent illness. Concerned about the side effects of conventional drugs, an English physician, Edward Bach, explored natural, gentler ways to alleviate emotional difficulties and psychological imbalances. Unfortunately, no controlled scientific studies are available to support their effectiveness. One reason is that it's difficult to measure the effects of flower essences with standard scientific methods. Practitioners have relied on case studies and anecdotal evidence.

Since Edward Bach's death, further development of the flower essence repertory has been carried on by his protégés in England and the United States. Bach and other flower remedies require patience. They are not quick fixes like tranquilizers or sleeping pills, but neither do they create physical dependence or have side effects. The subtle, gentle action of flower essences makes them safe for use in self-help for mild anxiety.

Bach and other flower essences can be purchased in concentrated form in many health food stores. Put 3 to 4 drops of the concentrate in a 1-ounce bottle of spring water. Place 4 drops under the tongue first thing in the morning, between meals, and before going to sleep. Up to six remedies may be combined and taken at one time, but the fewer mixed together, the better. Each of the different flower remedies is considered to be effective for a specific mental attitude or set of symptoms. Here are nine Bach flower remedies, followed by the symptoms of anxiety and fear for which they are used:

- Rock Rose: panic, terror, and nightmares
- Red Chestnut: excessive worry about the health and safety of loved ones
- Aspen: apprehension, dread, vague fears for no apparent reason
- Impatiens: impatient, anxious for a hasty recovery
- Star of Bethlehem: the shock of loss or bad news; great distress or fright following a trauma
- Clematis: dreamy, drowsy, and not fully awake; faintness or out-of-body sensations
- Larch: persistent low-level anxiety
- Cherry Plum: fear of losing your mind or going crazy; irrational persistent thoughts of hurting yourself or suicidal impulses
- Mimulus: specific known fears; shyness, timidity, indecisiveness

Note: Flower remedies and their applications are presented for interest only and with no claims of effectiveness. As there is no published scientific research, support for these is mostly anecdotal. They are not a substitute for psychotherapy, nor are they meant to treat an anxiety disorder that requires medical attention. If symptoms persist or you feel out of control, immediately consult a doctor or other qualified health professional.

RESCUE REMEDY

One of the best-known flower remedy formulas for stress relief is sold under brand names such as Rescue Remedy, Calming Essence, Five Flower Formula, and Nature's Rescue. Dr. Edward Bach developed this formula by blending five of his flower remedies together—Impatiens, Clematis, Rock Rose, Cherry Plum, and Star of Bethlehem. Rescue Remedy is the most frequently used combination of all the Bach flower remedies. It is used worldwide as first aid for its calming effect on anxiety, grief, and trauma. It is used for such everyday stresses as tension headaches, temper tantrums, and stage fright. It is said to be helpful for anticipatory anxiety before taking a test, going to the doctor or dentist, or giving a speech. It may also be of assistance in an emotional crisis, such as trauma after an accident or grief over a loved one.

Rescue Remedy should never be used as a substitute for emergency medical evaluation and treatment. In addition, no scientific studies have documented the effectiveness of Rescue Remedy. When stress relief is needed, place 4 drops of Rescue Remedy under the tongue, directly from the bottle. You can also put 4 drops in a cup of warm water and sip it slowly every few minutes until the crisis abates. Rescue Remedy can be obtained at most health food stores. Keep the remedy closed tightly in its original container, and store away from sunlight and heat.

HOMEOPATHY

Through the like, disease is produced, and through the application of the like, it is cured.

—HIPPOCRATES

Homeopathy is a system of healing based on the principle "like cures like." *Homeo* means "similar" and *pathy* means "disease or suffering." Homeopathy is primarily a German medical tradition, with its roots in ancient Greece. Almost two-thirds of all homeopathic remedies are prepared from plant materials, including fruits, flowers, vegetables, roots, seeds, berries, and the bark of trees.

In homeopathy, symptoms are seen as a healthy response of the body to illness. Suppressing or removing symptoms by standard allopathic medicine is viewed as not treating the underlying cause of the disease. Homeopathy holds that a very small dose of "similars" is capable of inducing a healing response in an ill person with similar symptoms. The best example of this in American medicine is probably allergy shots, in which a very small amount of the allergic substance (known as the allergen) is injected into the allergic person to treat the allergic condition.

Homeopathic prescriptions are formulated by serial dilution and succussion (vigorous shaking). The majority of homeopathic remedies are at relatively low dilutions: 3X–30X, meaning that the mother tincture (1 mg per 10 cc) has been diluted out 3–30 times (taking 9 cc out and adding back 9 cc of water each time), with interval succussion.

Homeopathy strives to treat the whole person, rather than different specialists treating separate symptoms. In keeping with a holistic, natural view of medicine, the patient's emotional and spiritual aspects are considered just as important as the physical in achieving a cure. Homeopaths consult a *Materia Medicas* to determine the remedy that best matches the whole picture of the patient's symptoms. The choice of remedies is determined by taking a detailed case history to elucidate the patient's overall constitutional needs, not just the evident symptoms. Homeopathy is a safe and effective, though still controversial, system for treating transient anxiety and chronic stress.

Dr. Klaus Linde and other respected researchers, including Wayne B. Jonas, M.D., director of the Office of Alternative Medicine at the National Institutes of Health, thoroughly reviewed 89 placebo-controlled studies of homeopathic treatments reported in the medical literature. Their results were published in the September 20, 1997, issue of the acclaimed medical journal *Lancet*. Their meta-analysis of the data pooled from these 89 studies showed that homeopathic remedies were almost two-and-a-half times more effective than placebo.

Homeopathic remedies are derived not only from plants and herbs but also from animal and mineral sources. The following are some examples of remedies a homeopath might use, after taking a detailed case history, to match specific symptoms of stress and anxiety:

- Ignatia—worry, insomnia, fear, and emotional strain
- Gelsemium—stage fright, apprehension, trembling, and diarrhea
- Aconite—anxiety, throbbing headache, faintness, or dizziness
- Pulsatilla—insomnia, anxiety, fearfulness
- Arsenicum album—worry, exhaustion, and fatigue
- Coffea cruda—jittery nerves, racing thoughts, mental strain

For transient mild anxiety you can treat yourself with appropriate remedies that can be purchased in many health food stores. Two homeopathic remedies from Lehning Laboratories of France—Sleep Ease, a nonhabit-forming sleep aid, and Anti-Anxiety, for daytime stress—are especially popular in Europe, and are now distributed throughout the United States. Follow the directions on the label. Be sure to take homeopathic remedies at a separate time of day from other herbs and medications. It is also best if the mouth is free of food, coffee, tea, toothpaste, or mouthwash at the time of ingesting the remedy.

Many hundreds of American physicians and other licensed health care practitioners use homeopathy as an alternative medicine. If you are considering homeopathy as part of your treatment for anxiety, it would be best to consult a trained homeopath. Because the symptoms of anxiety can vary so widely from one person to another, working with someone experienced in homeopathy is preferable to attempting to self-treat with remedies available in health food stores. Do not discontinue any prescription drugs without consulting your doctor or a homeopathic physician.

HERBAL MEDICINES ARE A CATALYST OF NATURAL HEALING

Nature is the healer of disease.

—HIPPOCRATES

Healing comes from within, and it is your birthright. Herbal remedies are a catalyst for the innate power to heal anxiety. Just as you might choose to say grace before a meal, each time you take a botanical medicine you might affirm, "This herb is to heal my mind and body, and for my spiritual growth." You can trust your healing, for nature is now on your side.

Although you may be receiving guidance, advice, and suggestions from one or more health care professionals, your healing is fundamentally in your hands and heart. Most of all, have faith in the doctor who resides in you. It is also important that you form a safe, strong alliance with the health care provider you choose. You must decide among the various courses of treatment presented. Don't become a

sheep. Become educated. Ask questions. If your doctor suggests an herb or synthetic medicine, ask about benefits, risks,
and side effects. Make an informed decision, and follow
through on the treatment you choose.

Recognize and accept that plateaus will occur. The body
does not heal in a smooth, continuous fashion. It is natural
for your healing journey to consist sometimes of two steps
forward and one step back. Enjoy your healing, and don't be
discouraged. If you have suffered from stress and anxiety for
a long time, you may discover a confidence and inner peace
you have not known for years.

PART 3

NATURAL SELF-HEALING

Come forth into the light of things. Let nature be your teacher.

—WILLIAM WORDSWORTH

21

The Healing
Journey—Nurturing
Your Natural Self

*After a time of decay comes the turning
point. The powerful light that has been
banished returns.*

—I CHING

Herbal remedies are a powerful, practical means for healing
anxiety naturally. Anxiety, however, also signals a need to
change to a more healthful lifestyle. Health is much more
than the absence of dis-ease; it is a positive state of well-
being. The tools and techniques of the natural self-healing
program have been developed and refined over thirty years in
the practice of integrative psychiatry, alternative medicine,
and psychotherapy. You can start at any point, with any of
the strategies in Part 3, to immediately feel more inner peace
and personal power.

Where's the best place to start? That's up to you. "But,"
you may be wondering, "do I need to use all the natural self-
healing strategies to get results?" (This is a common perfec-

tionistic, all-or-none sign of anxiety.) Absolutely not. You can begin anywhere with whatever first interests you. The natural self-healing program provides tools and techniques that can be valuable, but how you do these exercises is equally important. These strategies are intended to make your life easier and more enjoyable, not more stressful and complicated. By making the simple yet significant improvements suggested in the pages ahead, you can get unstuck from a fearful rut and take control of your life, work, and relationships.

Healing stress and anxiety is a challenge for nearly everyone in our fast-paced "I want it done yesterday" world. Herbal medicines can be a wonderful start because they help you get rapidly back in touch with your natural self. But then you must make some changes in your habits and lifestyle to heal anxiety at the core. Natural self-healing does not involve an impractical return to some dreamt-of Shangri-la but offers insights and ideas, tools and strategies for a busy person like you. On the pages that follow, you'll find suggestions for greater well-being, not a rigid set of rules.

When you consider a particular new attitude or technique, ask yourself, "How do I feel about this suggestion?" Pay attention to the answers you get. Listen to the inner wisdom of your body as it expresses itself through signs of comfort or discomfort, alertness or fatigue. Make the choices that seem most natural for you—simple, comfortable, unforced, revitalizing. Watch the results. The intention is always to help you achieve a higher state of well-being with less struggle and strain.

Remember that everything counts; small decisions sometimes pay the largest dividends. For example, protecting yourself from interruptions while you are concentrating on work might restore some peace of mind at the office. A regular exercise program, reducing your caffeine intake, or creating a timeless bedroom can help you sleep more soundly. A few key choices can lighten your load and raise your spirit.

DO LESS, ACCOMPLISH MORE

Things which matter most should never be at the mercy of things which matter least.

—GOETHE

If you're feeling stressed, anxious, and worried, then you're already giving everything you've got just trying to stay afloat. What you need are practical, on-the-spot, real-life ways to:

- Accomplish more of your goals but not strain along the way
- Develop a calm, alert mind in the midst of a hectic schedule
- Sleep more deeply, night after night
- Maintain lifelong health and fitness without the hassles
- Develop emotional fitness to create more genuine inner peace and happiness
- Balance the competing demands of work and home
- Reconnect with your natural rhythms
- Correct misconceptions that can cause needless stress and anxiety
- Bring out your best during difficult times
- Burst through limiting fears to greater adventure and joy
- Acknowledge what you really feel and desire, underneath your anxiety
- Renew your spirit and discover greater meaning and purpose

You can learn to accomplish more of what matters most to you; to let go of unrealistic, guilt-loaded, time-pressured attempts to reduce stress and substitute simple strategies for natural well-being. To get more done by doing less is a cornerstone of natural self-healing. To accomplish this you must learn to live more in the *present*, not remain stuck in regret about the past or anxiety about the future. When you are caught in worrying about your past or future, there is never enough time, because your mind is trying to be in two places at once. Being more present allows you to enjoy a timeless, anxiety-free state. A relaxed presence allows you to visualize an optimum future and allows nature to do the organizing.

CONNECTING WITH
YOUR NATURAL SELF

The anxious self, grounded in the illusion of "I, me, mine," is ever vigilant for any real or imagined threat to survival. By this I mean not just your physical survival but the emotional survival of your self-concept: your opinions, pride, feelings, or the things with which you strongly identify. Holding on to your anxious self often robs you of peace of mind, satisfaction, and love. You contract your life energy around the anxious self that is supposed to protect you, but you wind up fearful and lonely instead.

The anxious self inhibits the spontaneous, free expansion that enables you to connect easily with your Natural Self. The Natural Self is connected to the vitally important issue of ego boundaries. If you feel you are an isolated person, disconnected from others and separate from nature, your inner state is anxious, contracted, and guarded. But if you can experience that your anxious, security-conscious self is not the deeper you, then your Self expands to all of nature.

Albert Einstein described the need for expanding self-awareness when he wrote: "A human being is part of the whole, called by us 'universe,' a part limited in time and space. He experiences his thoughts and feelings as something separate from the rest—a kind of optical delusion of his consciousness. This delusion is a kind of prison for us, restricting us to our personal decisions and to affection for a few persons nearest to us. Our task must be to free ourselves from this prison by widening our circle of compassion to embrace all living creatures and the whole nature in its beauty." William Blake put the matter succinctly: "If the doors of perception were cleansed, everything would appear to man as it is—infinite." Einstein's and Blake's visions suggest that when you are receptive to your Natural Self, you can transcend the optical delusion and prison of separation anxiety, and reconnect with the creative patterns of intelligence that govern the whole cosmos.

Most of us tie up enormous energy suppressing our feelings and trying to be someone we're not. There is a gulf between the anxious self that reacts to perceived threats, and the Natural Self that lies hidden within. The result of this split is an inner parade of doubt, irritation, and fear. As long as you let yourself remain burdened with these chronically anxious feelings, you inhibit your emotional freedom and diminish your joy and vitality.

The split between the natural and anxious selves begins when a child first gets scolded with the words "You're a bad child." What the parent means is that the child has done something that is unacceptable to the adult, but that's not what children hear and feel. They can't make the intellectual distinction between themselves and their behavior, so the scolding registers as "I'm bad," and the first crop of self-nullifying shame is sown.

In early adolescence it is very difficult not to succumb to the media image of the ideal, Miss Teenage America, perfect in every way. Instead of being encouraged to develop their unique talents and tastes, almost all adolescents measure themselves against a social ideal. They inevitably find themselves lacking in one or more categories. Even if they defiantly rebel, shame has once again scorched their innocent souls. This wave of shame is all the more painful because, as Joseph Chilton Pearce points out, "Adolescents sense a secret, unique greatness in themselves that seeks expression."

How about you? Were you upset about a facial feature—perhaps your nose or your chin? Maybe you thought you were too short or too tall. Were you happy with your figure? Did you think your breasts were too big? Too small? In the locker room, boys inevitably compare the size of their sexual organs, and some always leave feeling underendowed. The possibilities for self-deprecating shame and anxiety at this age are nearly endless. Strength, wit, intelligence, beauty, or athletic skill—any quality at all—is a potential source of anxiety about not measuring up, and therefore feeling worthless.

By the time most teens reach young adulthood, they have developed a two-tiered personality, and the inner joy and light of authenticity—freely and naturally being the person you are—is dimmed. This adolescent split in the personality peaks in the late teens. Reintegrating the public and private selves is a primary task of adulthood. Reconnecting with your deepest inner nature is important to healing anxiety, and feeling truly loved.

Most of us are only dimly aware of our innermost Natural Self. It communicates in the language of the heart and intuitive feelings, not in self-critical thoughts or anxious images. If you're like most people, you have been conditioned all your life not to trust your feelings. That conditioning explains in large part why the subtle voice of your Natural Self is so often ignored. The greater the discontinuity between your inner and outer selves, the more difficult it becomes to hear the quiet, gentle messages of your Natural Self.

To better understand the Natural Self, it may be helpful to know what it's not. It's not the part of your mind that engages in lengthy analysis. Your Natural Self speaks simply, not in complex arguments. It isn't the part of you that generates the internal chatter that sometimes makes decision-making difficult. The inner self can guide correct decision-making, often through a simple felt sense of yes or no. Your Natural Self is not your will and isn't subject to control; you can ignore it, but you can't force it. You have to listen to it and use your will to act on the insights you hear. Finally, your Natural Self is not the undulating flow of emotions. Though your innermost nature can communicate through feelings, it is better understood as that part of the self where feeling and thinking meet.

The more familiar you become with your Natural Self, the more you will appreciate the degree of personal power you have been ignoring. The Natural Self is able to know what we can't rationally explain. For example, for some people it can provide creative ideas that far exceed their limited estimates of their own intelligence; for others it can yield business hunches that result in remarkable payoffs; it can save time and energy by telling you exactly where to look for something you want; it can identify the smoothest path to achieve your goals.

Although your inner voice is naturally present, you must cultivate your ability to hear it. This may seem paradoxical, but it isn't. Walking is natural but must be learned. Speech is natural but also must be learned. So it is with your innermost voice. It's natural, but you must still learn how to use it. Contacting your Natural Self takes time, and a specific technique is helpful. Once you get good at the technique, however, you no longer need it. You can pause for a moment anywhere, anytime, and tune in to the messages from your deepest self. The better you get at this, the more you find yourself operating from your Natural Self all the time. At that point you are functioning with maximum personal power and vitality.

Here's how to contact your Natural Self. The process takes about fifteen to twenty minutes, so you need to set aside that much time to be alone in a comfortable and quiet place. Begin by closing your eyes and settling into a state of relaxation. Use any of the techniques in Chapter 24. After several minutes, when you're feeling at ease, begin to notice that you're able to sit back and observe the flow of thoughts and feelings in your mind and body.

Now you can clear an inner space, a quiet field of inner awareness that will allow you to get a felt sense of your Natural Self. As long as your mind is engaged in an almost constant inner chatter and preoccupied with all your daily concerns, you won't be able to hear the quiet messages from your deepest self. To create a quiet inner space, make a simple decision to set all your problems and worries aside. This doesn't require effort or forcing thoughts out of your mind. All that's really required is a decision, a clear intention to put your problems aside. Once you clear this inner space, you will settle deeper into yourself. You will begin to have a more intimate sense of your total bodily state. You may notice a tense muscle or a nagging worry, and that's OK. These subtle feelings indicate that you're clearing an inner space to learn what's really going on in the depths of your soul.

Now you're ready to choose a problem you want to work out. Choose any problem you like. It can be an emotional conflict or one having to do with a relationship. If you're doubtful about a business decision, you can choose to work on that. The point is: your Natural Self has much more information to bring to bear on any one of your problems than you normally give yourself credit for. Now you're accessing those deeper intuitions.

Gently bring your problem to mind. The trick is to neither focus on it too closely nor keep it at too great a distance. Let yourself be aware of the problem, and notice any feelings that begin to emerge. Don't hurry, and don't try prematurely to label what may begin to come up. Let the feeling grow on its own in response to the problem you chose to focus on. If the feeling shifts, follow it, don't force it. Attend to it as if watching an interesting movie. Gradually the feeling will take on a recognizable form.

The next step is to put your feeling into words. The feeling is giving you a new perspective on your problem, so don't be in a hurry to label it with stock phrases. Assume an experimental attitude. Words will come up. Gently match them against the feeling. If there's an approximate match, you'll have a deep, inwardly felt sense of rightness. There will be perhaps an "Aha." If the match is not good, the sense of rightness will be fuzzy. As you work with words to describe your feeling, use this sense of rightness as your guide. It's very similar to the sense of rightness you have when you adjust a crooked picture. When it's straight, you simply know it's right. So too with finding words to express your Natural Self. When it's clear, you'll feel it's right.

These are the outlines of the technique. The more you practice it, the better you'll understand it. Keep in mind that each step leads naturally to the next. If you try to exert too much control, you inhibit the whole process. Usually you'll find the entire experience pleasurable. If you're working on a difficult personal problem or repressed feeling, you may encounter a few rough spots. Go easy with any rough emotions that come up. Don't try to analyze them. Don't push them away either. If you let repressed feelings come to the surface, you'll find a great sense of relief. The repressed pain of old emotional wounds can dissolve in one big flow of feeling. All at once an inner block dissolves; perhaps you'll experience some tears. Afterward you'll have a new sense of emotional freedom and inner peace.

Until you become practiced at connecting with your Natural Self, you may have to use this technique regularly to get a clear answer to a particular problem. At times you may feel ambivalent about the messages you hear. Or you may get stuck on a feeling that won't move. Be easy with whatever comes up. Ask yourself, "What does this feeling mean?" Wait for a response. You'll probably find new feelings creeping into your awareness, changing your perception of the initial experience. If, after about fifteen minutes, you feel no sense of rightness or release from anything that has come up, let it be. Another time, when you feel more at ease, you can practice the technique again.

Uncertainty is fearful to the anxious self, which wants to control all experience. But a compulsive need for certainty leaves no room for a creative response. Experiencing the Natural Self means letting go and letting God surprise you. As you learn to connect with your Natural Self, life becomes more "re-creational," more creative and fun and free of worry, control, and strain. You gain more peace of mind as you accept the dance of the unexpected and the wisdom of uncertainty.

OVERCOMING *PSYCHOSCLEROSIS*— HARDENING OF THE PSYCHE

A major concern of modern medicine is arteriosclerosis, a hardening of the arteries that can result from chronic stress, poor diet, and inadequate exercise. There is a parallel psychological process for which I have coined the term *psychosclerosis*—a hardening of the mind, heart, and spirit. Just as arteriosclerosis constricts arteries and the flow of oxygen-rich blood, which can cause heart disease or a brain disorder, psychosclerosis constricts the flow of love, joy, and creativity. The resulting dis-ease and dis-order limit self-expression, erode vitality, and narrow the depth and capacity of feeling.

The parallels between arteriosclerosis and psychosclerosis are further revealing. While arteriosclerosis makes arteries stiff through calcification, psychosclerosis constricts emotions and makes thinking brittle. Arteriosclerosis can limit the joy of activity; psychosclerosis can take the passion out of life. The longer arteriosclerosis goes unchecked, the greater the risk of heart attack or stroke. Similarly, the longer psychosclerosis goes unchallenged, the greater the risk of a panic attack or agoraphobia.

PRINCIPLES OF
NATURAL SELF-HEALING

Natural self-healing techniques can reverse psychosclerosis just as physical exercises can undo arteriosclerosis. Each of these activities can either be enjoyable and healthful, if you pace yourself, or laborious and even self-defeating, if you try to accomplish too much too soon. Below are the major principles that apply to all the natural self-healing exercises in this part of the book.

- *You need to reevaluate your "comfort zone."* Many people get comfortable with feeling uncomfortable. Starting to feel more calm and peaceful may initially leave you feeling unusual, fearful, or strange. One of the first resistances you may experience to a natural self-healing exercise is "This isn't me; it doesn't feel natural." Expect this initial response because these "emotional fitness workouts" are developing new habits of feeling and self-concept. Think for a moment of how you felt when you first learned to ride a bicycle, ski, or play tennis. You probably felt a little

awkward, and the motions involved felt strange or even
artificial. You may have felt you would never develop the
grace and coordination required.

- *Repetition is the key to mastery.* With practice, hundreds of
repetitions later, a new athletic habit becomes automatic
and feels completely natural. It's the same with new emotions; at first they can feel strange or artificial. When you
practice an exercise to expand your behavioral repertoire,
you should expect to feel some initial awkwardness. As
you practice the exercise, you will soon begin to internal-
ize the new experience and value it. Ways of responding
that initially may seem mechanical will start to feel more
graceful, whether these involve better feelings about
yourself or relating more effectively to others. With
patience and practice, you will overcome any feelings of
discomfort and achieve mastery.

- *All psychological growth involves insight and behavior change.*
You can't expect to gain any benefits from this book by
rubbing its cover or placing it under your pillow. You must
put the insights and techniques into practice. In learning a
musical instrument or athletic skill, regular practice is the
key to success. Similarly, natural self-healing strategies and
exercises must be practiced regularly to achieve the results
you desire. Insight alone is rarely enough; you also need
behavior change. Keep in mind, however, that putting the
insights of this book into practice can also be fun, so enjoy
yourself as much as possible!

- *Stretch, don't strain.* Growth is a natural process that doesn't
need to be forced. An acorn doesn't strain to become an
oak tree; neither must you strain to grow. In a physical
fitness program, you would be cautioned against overdo-
ing it, which can lead to loss of motivation, discomfort,
even injury. As you heal anxiety, significant changes are
going to occur in how you feel about yourself. You won't

achieve the desired growth by pushing yourself to meet impossible standards. That kind of self-defeating pattern just ensures more anxiety. Set yourself up to win. If an exercise doesn't seem to be helping you achieve a result on a particular day, set it aside, and perhaps try it again another day. Be gently disciplined and firmly patient with yourself, as you would be in starting a Nautilus program or Jazzercise.

- *Accept opposites; welcome paradox.* Psychological growth involves the integration of seemingly opposite values (e.g., strength and tenderness, analysis and intuition, stability and flexibility, maturity and spontaneity). The paradox of growth is that you need to accept yourself as you are rather than strain to be what you are not or what you fantasize you ought to be. Healing anxiety with self-love and understanding can not only produce more lasting results but also make a vital difference in the effectiveness of your healing.

- *Difficulties and challenges will always arise.* There is no permanent victory in life; problems and challenges always arise. Growth is never in a straight upward line. It is more often an irregular path, two steps forward and one back. You may heal anxiety only to encounter a crisis that sets you back. There is a common tendency to revert to old habits under severe stress or a major loss. Don't despair if that happens. Use "backsliding" as a new opportunity to solidify and increase your progress. Crisis is an opportunity for further growth. Self-healing must be flexible and fluid, not a rigid, autocratic process.

22

From Pressure and Panic to Personal Power

*The deepest reality you are aware of is the
one from which you draw your power.*
—DEEPAK CHOPRA, M.D.

Is your internal motor running faster than the world around
you? Do you get impatient waiting for water to boil? When
the airline reservations line has you on hold, does the canned
music grate on your nerves? What if your lunch date shows
up half an hour late, and on the way back from lunch you find
that the automatic teller machine is out of order and the bank
clerk needs two approvals just to cash your check? Most people would gladly become less tense and rushed—if only they
had the time!

In a hectic world in which change and frenzy seem to be
the only constants, you may feel like a car racing out of control down a narrow mountain highway. How are you supposed to enjoy the ride or appreciate the scenery when you're
in constant danger of losing your grip and crashing over a
cliff? What is all this tension and rushing for? For many, it's

to be able to afford a heart attack, divorce, and psychotherapy for their children.

Most of us take on more than it's humanly possible to accomplish in any given day. Handling innumerable chores and crises at home, work, and in transit while also trying to pack in athletics, social activities, and fun, we hardly find time to come up for air. Sooner or later, as we try to cram more and more activities into less and less time, the body rebels. Human beings don't "suddenly" develop anxiety attacks. By the time anxiety strikes, there have been years of neglected clues to slow down, reexamine priorities, and listen to your body's signals.

You may have become so used to being under pressure, you don't remember what it's like to relax. Inactivity is what seems unpleasant or threatening to you. You try resisting, but your mind still races with things to do. You take a few moments of quiet with your family, and immediately an argument ensues. You take a day off from work and spend the entire time catching up on errands and chores. You have difficulty sleeping because you worry about your love life or work.

You may try to appear calm when you're under the gun, but your body knows the difference. Feigning tranquillity doesn't take the pressure off. Do you often find yourself thinking, "I don't have time," or "Time's running out," or referring to time lines and time pressures? Numerous opinion polls in the United States and Europe show that people complain more about lack of time than about lack of money or freedom. In recent years our collective sense of life's quickening pace— the feeling that time is growing shorter, more scarce—has become exaggerated. We're hurrying. We're straining to catch up. We're anxious about time. We're resentful about time. We feel helpless about time. We're time stressed.

The human body is not well suited to time struggle. Research strongly suggests that people who suffer from hurry sickness—the anxious feeling that there's never enough time—may be at increased risk of developing health problems such as high blood pressure and heart disease. Impatient clock-watching is also linked to hostility, resentment, and sudden cardiac death (an unexpected fatal heart attack).

The truth is that many of us waste enormous amounts of energy reacting automatically with frustration to even the most minor delays. We have thoughts such as "There's never enough time" and "What else can go wrong today?" Check to see if you have any of the following signs and symptoms of feeling chronically hurried, tense, and rushed:

- Taking on more when you are already overscheduled
- Feeling guilty relaxing when there's work to be done
- Feeling irritated by the shortcomings or demands of others
- Competing to show who's a harder worker
- Worrying when you have to delegate responsibility or ask for assistance
- Fearing that your success is due to speed and hard work rather than insight and creativity
- Becoming upset when you have to wait in line
- Wondering if people love you not for who you are but for what you do
- Suffering from tension headaches, muscle spasms, and indigestion
- Noticing what you fail to do instead of what you accomplish

If you notice feelings of time-related frustration day after day, it may be a warning sign that you have reached a potentially harmful level of hurry sickness.

TAKE FIVE

Try this simple test. Take an uninterrupted five minutes to sit comfortably, close your eyes, and let yourself relax. This is a time for idle enjoyment. If you open your eyes and see by your watch that the five minutes aren't over, close your eyes again and continue the test. *Now do this exercise before reading any further.*

Done? What happened? Did you find that the five minutes passed quickly or slowly? Were you mostly anxious, bored, and annoyed or calm and comfortable? The experience of time is highly variable. Though it is a cliché, time *does* seem to fly when we're having fun and to crawl when we have to do something unpleasant. If you're like most people, the five minutes passed slowly and you felt bored and restless. Did your thought stream sound like mental clamor, or were you able to enjoy the sound of silence? Perhaps your mind was filled with thoughts of all the things you have done or need to do. Perhaps you noticed some tension in your shoulders and neck. Perhaps you started worrying or feeling angry about what appeared to be a waste of time. These are all signals of tension and pressure.

Most time pressures are self-inflicted. Go through the list of the demands placed on you, and eliminate those you've needlessly created for yourself. Ask yourself the basic question "Do I really have to do this?" To reduce anxiety, you must make your health and well-being the number one priority. You need to reexamine your time commitments in order to restore vitality to your life. Ask yourself:

- "Does this meeting I've called have to take place?"
- "Do I have to cook for the dinner party tomorrow, or will my friends be just as happy if we order something from a restaurant?"
- "Do I belong to too many organizations?"

- "Do I have too many subscriptions to concert series and ball games?"
- "Do I have more social obligations than I can enjoy?"

Stop taking pride in how much you overwork. Ask yourself throughout the day whether what you are doing is your biggest priority or just more busy-ness. Rather than priding yourself on the number of hours you put in, use your creative ingenuity and plan wisely. It's more efficient to take a preventive measure to reduce stress and strain than to burn out.

PACE YOURSELF

Most of us have a tendency to take on a lot more in a given period of time than we can manage. Too often we plan a project without allowing enough time for things to go wrong (as they often do). An effective strategy is to create deadlines that allow an extra 20 percent of time for human error, delays, and unanticipated problems. If things go remarkably well, the worst that can happen is the pleasure and personal reward of finishing ahead of schedule.

Organize your work so that you can always enjoy calm. This is not as difficult as it sounds. The key is to be organized and to have a system for keeping track of your priorities. It helps to have four different files through which all your work flows. They should read Routine Work, Urgent, Think, and Work at Hand. Everything that comes across your desk should fall into one of the first three folders and remain there until you decide to move it to the position of work at hand. Once you start using this system, your work will take on a natural rhythm that will free you from unnecessary anxieties.

Become aware of your optimum rest/activity cycle. Just as you have a unique personality, you have an optimum work and play cycle that are likely to be different from anyone else's. Some people do their best work in the morning; others have an intense burst of concentration toward the end of the day; others have concentration bursts for brief intervals throughout the day. We call these periods of maximum alertness *prime times.* Once you understand your prime time, you can schedule your activities so that you'll tackle the important and challenging ones at your peak creative periods and relegate mundane activities to your low points.

Substantial evidence indicates that your prime time and optimum work cycle are biologically or even genetically determined. Trying to force yourself into an unnatural pattern (such as doing your most difficult work in the morning when you concentrate best in the afternoon) is a big mistake. You'll cause needless tension, your work will suffer, and you'll cheat yourself out of both enjoyment and creativity.

Take satisfaction in saying no. Sooner or later we all have to learn limits. We can't be all things to all people or try to do everything that comes along. We must choose what really matters to us, or outside demands will shape our lives.

Schedule your breaks with as much serious intention as you would a meeting with a top client. Too often we let problems at work push everything else aside. Relaxed time with loved ones deserves a high priority. Enjoying a leisurely walk in the park is as important as accumulating assets for tomorrow.

PROTECT YOURSELF
FROM INTERRUPTIONS

Nothing is more jarring to the nervous system than repeated interruptions when you're in the midst of concentrating on an important problem. One of the worst mistakes is to get into the habit of taking every phone call no matter what you're doing. A good way to handle the telephone is to concentrate your calls in one time segment, say between nine and ten in the morning or four and five in the afternoon. During that time you take all calls and return calls. You aren't being rude to refuse a call because you're busy. You're being wise.

AVOID FIVE O'CLOCK FRENZY

For peace of mind, we need to resign as general manager of the universe.

—LARRY EISENBERG

Many people waste so much time each day on unimportant tasks that they habitually fall short of their projected goals for the day. The result is a mad flurry of activity just before the bell. Both the product and the person suffer as a result. If you set realistic goals, don't waste time with people you don't need to see or tasks you don't need to do, and pace yourself, then you can wind down each workday with a smooth sense of accomplishment. Of course you won't always get everything done that you'd hoped, but each day will be successful because you will have accomplished the most important tasks or at least their most important parts. Routine work that you may not have completed can be left for a catch-up afternoon that you schedule once a week. Once you rid yourself of the five o'clock frenzy, not only will your work improve, but you'll also be a much more enjoyable person to be around.

RENEW YOUR CREATIVITY

I don't develop; I am.

—PABLO PICASSO

Hard work alone is never enough; you must listen to your inner voice to develop your creativity. When you are centered and not afraid of quiet reflection, you are less likely to run yourself ragged. Drive and hard work are necessary, but far more important are your creativity and enthusiasm. Over-work is a prime cause of anxiety and mental strain. Periods of rest and recovery each day and week are never a waste of time. Your brain and body will work better when you respect your biological rhythms of rest and activity. Anxiety constricts the pathways of creativity; relaxation reopens the channels.

The most valuable work you do may be done in five minutes of quiet—a brilliant idea, a pivotal decision, a simple solution. In those five minutes you can accomplish more than shuffling papers for twenty-four hours. If your daily schedule is so hectic that you can't take five minutes of rest when you need it, you are seriously shortchanging yourself. All life evolves and grows through cycles of rest and activity. The heart pumps and rests; we have cycles of day and night. Rest is the basis of dynamic activity.

Whenever you set a reasonable goal and meet it with time to spare, reward yourself with some time for re-creation. When you find creative ways to shorten your workload, delegate time-consuming activities, or eliminate unnecessary steps, you free up additional time and energy for intuition, pleasure, and inspiration.

GO WITH THE FLOW

Almost everyone has had the experience of starting work on a project and getting so immersed that they ignore time, fatigue, even where they are. Many hours later, when the task is completed, they become aware that they've been functioning at a unique high level where creative energies pour out effortlessly. Psychologists call this a state of *flow*.

This wonderful and productive state is not arbitrary. You can learn how to create it and then use it at will to accomplish a great deal of work in the shortest time. The key is learning what conditions trigger the inner shift from ordinary functioning to flow. For some people, quiet is necessary. Most people must be well rested. Time of day is almost always a key factor.

Flow is much more likely during your prime time than during a low period. Perhaps you need to be working at a particular desk or typewriter for flow to happen. There could be any number of critical conditions. Once you have learned what they are, you've made a major discovery. Flow is one of the basic means of doing less and accomplishing more. It's also a natural state of inner joy, even ecstasy.

VALUE YOUR TIME

When you are inspired by some great purpose, some extraordinary project, all of your thoughts break their bonds: Your mind transcends limitations, your consciousness expands in every direction, and you find yourself in a new, great and wonderful world. Dormant forces, faculties, and talents become alive, and you discover yourself to be a greater person by far than you ever dreamed yourself to be.

—PATANJALI

The need to value your time may seem too obvious to mention, and it would be if most people's actions reflected a true regard for their time. But they don't. All too often people fritter time away on unimportant activities; work overtime for an unappreciative boss who's taking advantage of their good nature and gullibility; sacrifice time that would be better spent enjoying their family rather than working late. Creating a new success profile absolutely requires that you seize control of your time and personal power.[1]

Above all, you must stop wasting time. One way is to ask a simple question: "Is this the most important thing I should be doing right now?" Don't worry about coming up with an answer. As soon as you ask this question, your inner voice will respond. Listen to what it says!

Spend a few minutes every day reviewing your priorities. Make a list of everything you want to get done each day, then rank the items in their order of importance. Your order of attack will change throughout the day as new situations come up, but setting up your priorities at the beginning of each day will be a helpful guide.

23

Active Living and Antistress Nutrition

*A good exercise prescription for the thirty
to fifty million mostly sedentary and unfit
Americans is "Turn off the television, get
up off your fanny, go out the door, and
move around a bit."*
—STEVEN N. BLAIR, M.D.

Research has shown that those people who are the most
resistant to stress and anxiety enjoy an active lifestyle. The
average American, however, watches television twenty-one
hours a week—an unprecedented chunk of time devoted to
staring at a glowing cathode-ray tube, requiring little energy
and virtually no activity. What is an active lifestyle? An
active lifestyle has five elements:

1. Enough stretching, twisting, reaching, and bending to
   maintain flexibility and elasticity
2. At least two hours of standing per day
3. Fifteen to twenty minutes daily of moderate aerobic exercise

4. Exertion of moderate physical effort once or twice daily, thus maintaining your strength and energy

5. Life-extending, stress-protecting nutrition

To meet these requirements, you don't have to make major changes in your daily routine. In fact, you may be surprised at how little you have to do to shift from a sedentary to an active, healthful lifestyle.[1]

REGULAR EXERCISE

Those who think they have no time for bodily exercise will sooner or later have to find time for illness.
—EDWARD STANLEY, EARL OF DERBY, 1873

Regular exercise, especially aerobics, can provide a powerful antidote to stress and anxiety. Research indicates that the happiest, healthiest people, at every age, are those who exercise regularly. Here are a variety of activities you can use to get more exercise throughout the day.

• Walk at least ten minutes from work to eat your lunch—so that after eating you can enjoy a ten-minute walk back. Walk up a flight or more of stairs rather than taking an elevator three to four times a day. When at a shopping mall, walk up the escalators instead of riding like a mannequin. A Harvard study demonstrated that a half-hour walk can even increase your IQ. Take time at home to walk with loved ones, friends, or the dog. Shovel snow from the sidewalk or driveway, take out the trash, rake some leaves, play sports with neighborhood children, or pedal on a stationary bicycle while watching television or talking on the telephone.

- Feel ready to yell at someone? Instead you could hit a punching bag for ten minutes or release some of your frustrations by gliding through a hundred strides on a cross-country ski machine.
- Play doubles tennis, play a game of Frisbee, or shoot some baskets. Join a walking club. Whenever possible make this an enjoyable family time—when your loved ones or friends join you in the activities.
- Run, swim, or bicycle for twenty minutes.

You don't really have to try very hard to get the exercise you need. It's just a matter of changing your attitudes and orientation from sedentary to active. But make sure your exercise is enjoyable; if you're straining or pushing yourself, it will not be as beneficial in reducing anxiety.

GETTING STRONGER

A strong body makes the mind strong.
—THOMAS JEFFERSON

Dr. Elmer Greene of the Menninger Clinic in Topeka, Kansas, hailed the revolution in mind-body medicine in 1970 when he wrote, "Every change in the physical state is accompanied by an appropriate change in the mental-emotional state." By physically strengthening yourself, you can also get emotionally stronger and mentally tougher. Building and maintaining muscle tone is an integral part of natural self-healing to diminish fear and anxiety. With healthy, strong muscles, your mental-emotional state will also be stronger and more resistant to stress.

It doesn't take long to produce results with strength training. According to the latest guidelines from the American College of Sports Medicine, all it takes for solid, progressive strength-training results is a total of fifteen minutes of strengthening exercises three or four times a week—using weight machines or body weight calisthenic exercises.

During each strengthening exercise, use good posture, smooth controlled movements, and even breathing. Don't hold your breath while exercising, since this may cause an unhealthy rise in blood pressure. Breathe evenly and steadily. Maintain balanced posture throughout every movement—don't arch your back or use any sudden twisting motions. Listen to your body. A mild burning sensation is usually acceptable discomfort; pain of any kind is not.

A slight soreness the next day is common when beginning to exercise. If you feel any pain during a particular movement, stop immediately. Consult your physician with any questions. Since safety and proper form are very important in strength-building exercises, consider getting some face-to-face professional guidance from a qualified fitness instructor. A session or two to learn effective workout techniques and to design a sensible program may be all you need.

Of course, getting stronger should not be confined to the gym. Other activities can provide a brief period of muscular exertion. For example:

- Carry two bags of groceries from the car at the same time.
- Open a vacuum-sealed jar. Don't bang the lid with a knife until you have tried two or three times with all your might first.
- If you have small children, lift them over your head a few times. You're helping yourself, and they'll love it.
- Move some furniture, change a tire, lift a bag of fertilizer, or do some other strenuous activity around the house.

FLEXIBILITY

Health is aliveness, spontaneity, gracefulness, and rhythm.
                              —ALEXANDER LOWEN, M.D.

Stress, anxiety, and worry cause your muscles to contract, leading to chronic tension. Many of us walk around in
a constant state of isometric tension, pushing against ourselves to restrict the natural flow of energy. The muscular
contraction caused by stress and anxiety can result in a tense
neck, sore back, tight jaw, or raised shoulders. Regular practice of yoga and tai chi can help you develop a flexible mind
and body and relieve tension. Stretch; don't strain. Here are
several of the easiest do-it-anywhere stretching exercises:

- *Back stretch:* Lie on the floor and get comfortable on your
  back. Now sit up, extending your hands above your head.
  Reach toward the ceiling and feel the energy streaming
  up from the base of your spine toward your head and into
  your arms. Now bend forward, stretching toward your
  toes until you feel a warm tingling sensation in your
  lower back. Breathe easily and feel the warmth of the
  stretch. Hold this position for a count of ten. Then lie
  back down and rest.
- *Pelvic rotation:* Standing up, set your feet a shoulder width
  apart. Relax and place your hands on your hips. Breathe
  deeply, and slowly move your hips around in a wide circular motion. Try not to lead with your shoulders or head,
  but instead allow your pelvis to initiate all the motion.
  Rotate five times to the right and then five times to the
  left.
- *Neck rotation:* Sit upright in a firm chair. Relax and
  breathe deeply, then let your chin drop slowly toward
  your chest. Continue to breathe normally while you

slowly roll your head to the right so that your right ear moves toward your shoulder. Then slowly return to the original position with your chin dropped toward your chest. Try five rotations to the right, then five to the left. You will unlock your neck, upper back, and shoulders.

- *Pelvic rock:* Lie on your back and relax. Then slowly draw up your knees until your feet are flat on the floor. Breathe normally and relax. Next, press your tailbone against the floor to create a small arch in your back. Then slowly rock your pelvis so that your back is pressing against the floor. Now repeat this playful rocking motion five to ten times. Enjoy the energy in your legs, hips, and back.

- *Spinal roll:* Lie comfortably on your back, and extend your arms out from your shoulders with your palms down. Relax, breathe deeply, and pull your knees up toward your chest to a comfortable position. Now roll your head to the right while rolling your hips to the left until your legs are resting on the floor. Rest, breathe, then turn your head to the left while rolling your legs to the right until they rest together on the floor. Repeat this exercise five times.

- *Forward bend:* Stand erect, breathe deeply, and raise your hands above your head. Continue breathing easily while you slowly bend forward until your hands are dangling toward the floor. Don't bounce or strain to touch the floor. Let your attention go to the stretching in your legs and lower back. Feel the tingly warmth, relax, and breathe. Now slowly return to the upright position.

Finish off a set of these exercises with a few minutes of relaxation. Lie on the floor on your back, close your eyes, breathe deeply, and enjoy your rejuvenating rush of energy. Do these stretches when winding down in the evening or whenever you feel like a few minutes of relaxation.

An active approach to getting dressed in the morning can help you maintain your flexibility and elasticity:

- Before you put on your suit or dress, move your arms up, back, and around in a circular motion once or twice. Roll your head around and limber up your neck.
- While you're getting dressed, exaggerate your motions a bit. Turn your torso once far to the right and once again to the left.
- Stand up and bend over to put on your socks and tie your shoes.

Take opportunities to stretch and bend during the day. During the midafternoon break, you can stretch your neck by slowly rolling your head three times to the left, then three times to the right. You can give your torso a good stretch by sitting forward in your chair and twisting as far as you can in both directions to look behind you. Bending over to touch your toes even while seated in a chair will be good for your back, and standing up and then bending to touch your toes will be even better. Your arms and shoulders can benefit just by reaching as far as you can above your head, one arm at a time.

GARDENING IS GOOD MEDICINE

You don't need a green thumb to benefit from horticultural therapy. Gardening, one of the oldest healing arts, is receiving serious medical attention. In 1812 Dr. Benjamin Rush, a signer of the Declaration of Independence and founding father of the American Psychiatric Association, described the use of gardening to help his patients. Today patients at over three hundred U.S. hospitals are discovering that growing plants is a powerful natural medicine for emotional and physical healing. The American Horticultural Therapy Association, in Gaithersburg, Maryland, has close to nine hundred members.

People have a natural healing response to gardening with herbs, plants, flowers, and shrubs. From designing a garden to making preparations for planting, from pulling weeds to pruning and mowing, horticulture can help attune you to nature's rhythms and your own.

The growing demand for medicinal herbs such as *Hypericum*, milk thistle, and chamomile has led to a renaissance of backyard, and even window box, herb gardening. Small herbal farms are experiencing the "sweet smell of success" at farmers' markets throughout the United States. Whether you decide to turn herb gardening into a sideline business or simply enjoy going back to nature with Martha Stewart, growing *Echinacea* or California poppy can often be healing in itself.

ENJOYING NATURAL BEAUTY

Scientific studies indicate that when individuals view beautiful natural scenes—waterfalls, sky, trees, flowers, or green plants—they often feel reduced anxiety and can relax more easily. They are also less likely to have negative thoughts or experience stress. You might include some simple yet enticing changes of scenery on your daily work breaks. Examples: walking in your favorite nearby park, gazing at fish swimming back and forth in an aquarium, looking out your window at nearby trees or flowers, watching clouds form and swirl against the sky, enjoying the antics of birds or squirrels in a stand of trees.

If your work limits you to urban environs, consider taking a vacation to explore nature's beauty—canyons, forests,

snow-covered mountains, waterfalls, sandy beaches, or mead-
ows brimming with wildflowers. When people view beautiful
natural scenes, they report much higher levels of positive
energy and friendliness and a reduction of fear. Views of
lakes, ponds, streams, trees, and flowers produce lower levels
of stress arousal and higher alpha brain waves, a state associated with calm alertness.

FEED YOUR BRAIN

A poor diet plus vitamins is still a poor diet.
—ART ULENE, M.D.

Nutritional deficiencies are common among people who
are susceptible to stress and anxiety. To maintain active living,
you require a high-complex-carbohydrate, low-fat, moderate-
protein diet. Many national health organizations now advise
moving toward a vegetarian diet (including whole grains,
beans and legumes, fruits, vegetables, and low-fat or nonfat
dairy products) or a semivegetarian diet (a vegetarian diet
plus limited amounts of skinless poultry or fish and little if
any beef or pork).

A healthful, stress-protecting diet includes a wide array
of fresh seasonal fruits and vegetables, whole grains (eaten as
breads, pasta, side dishes, and in soups or casseroles), a variety of legumes (beans, peas, and lentils), low-fat or nonfat
dairy products, and limited amounts of nuts, seeds, eggs, fish,
and lean poultry. In a study at the University of Kuopio, Fin-
land, 38 percent of new vegetarians reported feeling more
alert and vigorous and less stressed and fatigued after seven
months. Fresh, whole organic foods are the best source of
nutrients. Vitamin supplements alone cannot provide the
nutrition you need for good health.

THE BEST NATURAL PRODUCTS

Let food be your medicine.

—HIPPOCRATES

The best natural products you can take are without a doubt fruits and vegetables. Indeed, one of the smartest, quickest, and simplest ways to stressproof yourself is to eat five to nine servings of fruits and vegetables each day. According to the latest scientific and medical research, fresh fruits and vegetables offer your brain and body more than just fiber and complex carbohydrates. In fact, there are a whole range—perhaps thousands in all—of *phytochemicals* (*phyto* is derived from the Greek word for "plant") and other unique protective factors in these powerhouse natural foods. Some of these antiaging, antidisease chemicals are *limonenes* in citrus fruits, *indoles* and *isothiocyanates* in broccoli, *flavones* in dried beans, *genistein* in soybeans, and *flavonoids* in nearly every fruit and vegetable. A growing number of scientists are contending that the disease-preventing potential of these phytochemicals may be even greater than that of vitamins.

For fruits and vegetables, fresh is usually best. But if you just don't like these foods raw or can't find good-quality produce, there's no reason not to consume cooked, frozen, canned, or juiced fruits and vegetables, because they may still retain much of their value. Fruits and vegetables help neutralize free radicals—highly unstable, reactive "pyromaniac" molecules that can bind to and destroy cellular compounds. Damage from free radicals contributes to the increased incidence of degenerative diseases among those who suffer from chronic stress and anxiety.

As discussed on page 50, one of the negative consequences of excessive stress is increased production of free radicals in the body. Free radicals are also created in the body by exposure to sunlight, X rays, ozone, tobacco smoke, car exhaust, and other environmental pollutants. Free radicals set off chain reactions that convert fats to peroxides, which produce more and more free radicals. This leads to a destructive effect that biochemists call a *cascade*. Beyond altering biochemical compounds, corroding cell membranes, and killing cells outright, the predominant damage caused by free radicals may be to mutate DNA. Scientists increasingly believe that the destructive power of free radicals may play a significant role in the development of cancer and heart disease. Fruits and vegetables are rich in the antioxidants that prevent free radical damage.

AVOIDING TOXIC CHEMICALS IN FOOD

The destructive effects on health of toxic agricultural chemicals, such as pesticides, herbicides, and fungicides, are well documented. Many of these toxic chemicals are so dangerous to human health that they are banned in this country by the Food and Drug Administration. Instead, U.S. manufacturers are selling them to foreign countries, where they're sprayed on crops that in some cases are then exported for consumption in America. According to recent estimates, an average of twenty-seven tons of pesticides leave the United States for shipment overseas every hour of the day, and this figure doesn't include the huge quantities of pesticides transported by truck and train to Mexico and Canada.

Support legislation that will ensure quality food for the consumer. Agrichemical use could be dramatically reduced through the widespread application of organic farming methods. Also, mandate the labeling of genetically engineered foods. Consumer demand will create a healthier food supply.

Buy certified organically grown produce that is free of toxic chemicals.

Always wash your fruits and vegetables to reduce your exposure to potentially harmful chemical residues. Washing produce, with a drop of mild dishwashing soap added to a pint of water, can help remove some, but not all, of the chemical residues as well as any dirt and harmful bacteria. Use a vegetable brush, rinse off completely, and choose a soap product that isn't loaded with dyes and other chemicals.

CARBOHYDRATES AND SUGAR

All you see I owe to spaghetti.

—SOPHIA LOREN

Eating carbohydrate-rich snacks can reduce feelings of impatience and stress. During times of stress and anxiety, the brain rapidly depletes its supply of serotonin. A high-carb meal or snack fuels the production of this neurotransmitter and may help restore a calm mind and relaxed emotions, a state that can last for up to three hours.

Pasta, bagels, whole-grain bread, fruits, vegetables, rice, baked potatoes, and rye crackers are examples of foods high in carbohydrates that can help you feel less stressed and more at ease. These complex, fiber-rich starches have also been shown to reduce body fat. High-carb snacks in midmorning and midafternoon, such as an English muffin topped with your favorite all-fruit preserve, or a low-fat muffin, help keep your blood sugar steady all day. Healthy snacks contribute to weight loss by keeping your metabolism running at peak efficiency.

Unfortunately, the standard grain choices for most families are still white, bleached, all-purpose wheat flour and polished white rice, even though traditional whole-grain recipes offer a wide range of delicious tastes and textures. You can benefit by expanding the variety of dietary whole grains you consume to include cooked or baked foods that are high in amaranth, barley, brown rice, buckwheat, bulgur (cracked wheat), corn, millet, oats, quinoa, rye, triticale, and whole wheat. Fresh-baked breads and rolls, pasta, tortillas, and low-fat or nonfat muffins, biscuits, cereals, chips, crackers, and cookies are nutrient-rich foods that can play a valuable role in a health-enhancing diet. Your carbohydrates, however, should come primarily from fruits and vegetables. Don't overeat carbohydrates that come from whole grains, because these stimulate insulin production, which can make you feel sluggish.

Diets high in refined white sugar have been linked to increased anxiety. Excess sweets can cause a buildup of lactic acid in the bloodstream, which can lead to nervousness, tension headaches, and panic attacks in susceptible individuals. Foods and drinks that are high in sugar can contribute to premenstrual syndrome. Refined white sugar along with its counterparts (dextrose, fructose, maltose, and cane syrup) are found in processed foods, so read labels carefully. It makes sense to lower your consumption of sweeteners and highly sweetened foods to help reduce anxiety.

When your blood sugar is low, situations that normally don't hassle you can turn into stressful events. Low blood sugar, caused in many people by skipping meals or eating sweets instead of carbohydrate-rich snacks, causes the release of adrenaline in your bloodstream, which makes your anxiety higher and your temper shorter. Eat fresh, natural, or minimally processed foods such as whole grains, fruits, vegetables, and legumes. The latter food groups are digested slowly and efficiently, providing a steady source of energy without the biochemical roller-coaster effect of concentrated sugars. These are also excellent sources of vitamins, minerals, and other protective nutrients.

VITAMIN AND
MINERAL SUPPLEMENTS

In addition to a good diet, it makes sense to take a broad-spectrum vitamin-mineral supplement. In particular, a healthy intake of the B-complex vitamins is important for keeping stress and anxiety at bay:

- Thiamin (vitamin B_1) deficiency can include such symptoms as fear, insomnia, confusion, and mood swings. Good sources of vitamin B_1 are whole grains, fresh peas, beans, oranges, and fortified cereals and baked goods.
- Riboflavin (vitamin B_2) helps to transform amino acids into neurotransmitters. Good food sources of vitamin B_2 are broccoli, spinach, milk, yogurt, poultry, and fish.
- Niacinamide (vitamin B_3) is also vital to nervous system function. Good sources are tuna, chicken breast, and fortified breads and cereals.
- Pantothenic acid (vitamin B_5) is also known as the "antistress" vitamin, because it's one of the nutrients that fuels the adrenal glands. Good food sources of pantothenic acid are mushrooms, salmon, peanuts, and whole grains.
- Vitamin B_6 is needed by the body to manufacture serotonin, a neurotransmitter that plays a significant role in regulating anxiety. Good food sources of vitamin B_6 are bananas, avocados, chicken, eggs, soybeans, whole wheat, and walnuts. People with Parkinson's disease who take levodopa should not take vitamin B_6 supplements.
- The safest, most convenient way to make sure you are getting all of the above B vitamins is to take a quality B-complex supplement twice a day.
- Vitamin B_{12} deficiency can cause psychological difficulties, neurological problems, insomnia, and anemia. Your doctor can test you for this as well as for other nutri-

tional deficiencies. Good food sources of vitamin B_{12} are clams, crab, tuna, and salmon. You might need to take B_{12} under your tongue or as a shot because this vitamin is often absorbed poorly from the diet.

Vitamin E is a fat-soluble antioxidant that neutralizes free radicals. In addition to playing a significant role in the prevention of cancer, coronary heart disease, and cataracts, vitamin E is able to slow the progression of Alzheimer's disease, according to a 1997 study reported in the *New England Journal of Medicine*. Vitamin E, as alphatocopherol, was given at a dosage of 200 international units daily to 341 patients for 440 days. Vitamin E was just as effective as selegiline, a pharmaceutical drug used in the treatment of Alzheimer's.

Good food sources of vitamin E are vegetable and nut oils, including soybean, safflower, corn, and wheat germ. It's hard to get therapeutic levels of vitamin E, however, just from eating these foods. By regularly taking vitamin E supplements, you can cut the risk of heart attack by about 40 percent and prevent the development of several degenerative processes associated with aging. The benefits of vitamin E can be obtained with daily doses of up to 400 international units. There are no serious side effects at that level, though diarrhea and headaches have been reported. Vitamin E supplements should not be taken by those with vitamin K deficiency or with known blood coagulation defects or by those receiving anticoagulation therapy.

A daily mineral supplement is also helpful. Alcohol and caffeine, and even stress, can remove magnesium from your system. Copper, chromium, and manganese play roles in your body's production of neurotransmitters. Researchers at the University College of Swansea in Wales found that people who took supplements of 100 mcg of selenium a day felt less anxiety, fatigue, and depression than those who did not. If you are a strict vegetarian, you must be especially careful that your mineral supplement contains selenium. The only good food sources for selenium are lobster, crab, clams, and cooked oysters. Whole grains and Brazil nuts have small amounts of selenium.

NATURAL BRAIN BOOSTERS

A decline in brain power is not inevitable as you age. In addition to the marvels of *Ginkgo biloba* extract, which enhances the flow of blood and oxygen to the brain, other natural supplements show promise as brain-savers:

- Phosphatidylserine (PS), a compound that is highly concentrated in brain cells, helps protect these cells against the harmful effects of the stress hormone cortisol. PS in brain cells is gradually replaced by cholesterol, a "hardening of the neurons" that can cause memory to fade with age. Research conducted at Stanford and Vanderbilt universities showed that taking a PS supplement helped improve memory in just one month. PS was formerly derived only from cattle brains, but a PS product made from soybeans is now available. Take 100 mg three times a day for the first month, and then lower to 100 mg of PS daily for a maintenance dose.
- Phosphatidylcholine (PC), found in lecithin, is needed to synthesize acetylcholine, a neurotransmitter vital to memory. Take 1000 mg three times a day.
- Docosahexaenoic acid (DHA), a long-chain fatty acid, is essential for normal brain function. Studies have linked low levels of DHA to reduced concentration, memory loss, and visual impairment. Good food sources are omega−3-rich fish (salmon, albacore, halibut, and sardines), soy, and eggs. Take 1000 to 1500 mg daily.

- Coenzyme Q10 (CoQ10), a potent antioxidant, is involved in energy production mechanisms in cells. It can help improve blood circulation to the brain, increase energy, and protect the heart. Take 100 to 200 mg daily. Give CoQ10 a good two-month trial.
- Acetyl-L-carnitine (ALC), an amino acid, can improve mood, aid memory, and increase energy. Take 1500 to 2000 mg daily.

Good nutrition and exercise are vital to giving the brain a boost. Regular exercise pumps more oxygen-rich blood to your brain. Sound nutrition provides the building blocks for the optimum growth of neurons. Of course, if you do experience a sudden or drastic loss of memory, please see your doctor immediately. It could be the result of a treatable condition such as high blood pressure, diabetes, or a benzodiazepine or other drug you might be taking.

HORMONE REPLACEMENT

There has been research on the use of natural hormones to boost the aging brain. Dehydroepiandrosterone (DHEA) is produced by the adrenal glands and gonads. Optimum levels of DHEA occur around age twenty, after which they gradually decline. By age seventy, DHEA levels may have dropped to a fraction of what they were at twenty. DHEA is important to health as a hormone regulator and as a precursor to estrogen and progesterone. DHEA supplements, when appropriate, can improve sleep, memory, and the ability to cope with stress.

Pregnenolone is a hormone produced in the brain and adrenal cortex from cholesterol. Pregnenolone is a building block from which DHEA and other hormones are produced. By about age forty-five, pregnenolone begins to progressively decline. This hormone enhances vitality, mood, memory, concentration, and other cognitive functions. Your doctor can order laboratory tests to check the levels of both pregnenolone and DHEA. If supplementation with either DHEA or pregnenolone is appropriate, it should be done only under medical supervision.

Various studies have shown at least a 45-percent lower risk of Alzheimer's disease among women who take estrogen replacement therapy after menopause. Estrogen is effective in stimulating the growth of neurons, or brain cells, and blunts stress-related cortisol release. There is strong scientific evidence that supports personalized, minimum-dosage estrogen replacement therapy, in consultation with your doctor.

A possible alternative is to consume foods rich in *phytoestrogens*, plant estrogens. Phytoestrogenic foods and herbs can help to relieve hot flashes, as well as anxiety and irritability. Soybeans, flaxseeds, kale, yams, millet, bok choy, and mustard greens are high in phytoestrogens. Herbs rich in estrogen-promoting compounds are black cohosh and Asian ginseng. It makes sense for perimenopausal women to increase their intake of legumes, vegetables and herbs containing phytoestrogens. More research is needed to determine whether plant estrogens can replace pharmaceutical estrogen (principally Premarin), for the prevention of osteoporosis and heart disease after menopause.

REDUCING CAFFEINE

Caffeine is a stimulant. People who are susceptible to anxiety are often more sensitive to caffeine. Too much coffee can trigger panic attacks, heart palpitations, and a generalized anxiety disorder. One of the simplest ways to reduce anxiety is to avoid overstimulating yourself with caffeine. Caffeine is found not only in coffee but also in tea, cola soft drinks, chocolate, over-the-counter medications (such as Excedrin), and weight control pills. According to a 1992 study in the *New England Journal of Medicine*, even moderate amounts of caffeine consumed during the week can leave you feeling out of sorts if you suddenly withdraw from the caffeine on Saturday and Sunday. Two cups of coffee can be enough to trigger intense anxiety and even panic attacks.

If you suffer from insomnia, avoid coffee, tea, and other caffeinated drinks within four or five hours of bedtime. Not only will caffeine keep you stimulated and awake, but it also acts as a diuretic that will increase the need to urinate during the night.

Caffeine is also addictive. Withdrawal symptoms include headache, decreased mental alertness, irritability, and fatigue. Caffeine should be gradually reduced over the course of many weeks to minimize these symptoms. Consider switching to herbal teas without caffeine, such as chamomile or peppermint. Or if you are looking for a mild amount of caffeine, switch to Japanese green tea, which is also an excellent general tonic.

COOLING THE SMOKING HABIT

Nicotine is one of the most addictive substances known. Its stimulant effect on the nervous system can contribute to anxiety in smokers as well as in users of snuff or chewing tobacco. Heavy exposure to secondhand smoke also has this risk. Research indicates that smoking one pack of cigarettes a day for thirty years or more can shorten one's life span by eight years. Cigarette smoking is the single most preventable cause of cancer, heart disease, and stroke. In addition to nicotine addiction, psychological factors play an important role in smoking. Some people smoke to try to control anxiety, "nerves," and social fears. Others use cigarettes to fight the boredom of getting stuck in traffic or to facilitate relaxation on a date.

Face your nicotine addiction intelligently. For the first seven to ten days after you quit, you will experience withdrawal. This means you should expect to be nervous, edgy, irritable, and tense. This also means that you should not try to quit during a pressure-filled time, such as before exams or an approaching deadline at work. When you are ready to quit smoking, consult your doctor. The American Cancer Society has an excellent smoking cessation program.

Recent research has shown that smokers are three times more likely to be depressed than nonsmokers. If the underlying depression is not treated, quitting smoking can be difficult if not impossible. The antidepressant and antianxiety effects of *Hypericum* are valuable for treating smokers who are depressed and wish to quit. Valerian and kava can help to reduce the agitation experienced during nicotine withdrawal. Taking a synthetic drug may also help smokers kick the habit. A recent study showed that the prescription antidepressant Zyban (bupropion) helped 25 percent of those who used it to quit smoking for at least a year. This drug helped more smokers quit for four weeks or more than Habitrol, nicotine transdermal patches.

Of course, people are prone to becoming addicted to other substances or activities in an effort to self-medicate or distract themselves from anxiety: food, sex, gambling, alcoholism, and drug abuse. More research is needed on the uses of herbal medicines in the treatment of addictions.

NATURAL HEALTH: THE POWER OF PREVENTION

Too many Americans suffer from poor health. Research published in 1996 in the *Journal of the American Medical Associa-*

tion documented that 45 percent of the United States pupula-
tion, over 100 million people, suffer from at least one chronic
disease.[2] America has the highest per capita health care costs
of any nation, spending almost one trillion dollars on medical
care. Yet the United States also has some of the worst health
statistics of any industrialized nation. Estimates indicate that
if the current trend prevails, the U.S. will spend 19 percent of
its gross domestic product (two trillion dollars) on medical
care in the year 2000. Thus far, cost containment strategies,
including managed care, have failed to stop the growth.

Why is the U.S. medical system such a cost-effectiveness
disaster? The answer is that our health care system is really a
"disease-care" system—it focuses on the management of
ilnesses rather than on the prevention of disease and the promotion of health. But the vast majority of our national health
is influenced by factors over which this diseasd-based
approach has little control—sucha as stress, nutrition, physical and emotional fitness, societal problems, and environmental toxins. Recent research shows that 50 percent of deaths
and 70 percent of disease in America are self-inflicted, caused
by an epidemic of unhealthy habits, including stressful
lifestyles, improper diet, inadequate exercise, smoking, and
alcohol and drug abuse.

In addition to serious illness, there is a virtual epidemic
of minor complaints. It is estimated that anxiety, headache,
lower back pain, gastrointestinal distress, chronic fatigue, and
other stress-related symptoms account for 80 percent of all
visits to family doctors. The amount of radio and television
time devoted to the advertising of nonprescription pain
relievers, decongestants, antacids, laxatives, and soporifics is
an obvious indication of how widespread the epidemic of
stress-related complaints has become.

The vast majority of disease is preventable. Yet only 1
percent of our health sector budget is used to avoid disease,

while 99 percent is spent to treat ilness after it occurs. Our individual and national focus must shift from disease care to true health care. These programs include prevention-oriented health education, including strategies to modify unhealthy behaviors and the use of prevention-oriented natural medicines. Recent studies indicate that specific programs of preventive health care avert disease before it arises and produce large cost savings:

- A ten-year study by the University of Michigan at Steelcase Corporation reported that systematic programs of diet, exercise, and stress reduction, when targeted for subjects in high health-risk categories, reduce total health care costws by 46 percent.[3]
- A program designed by Dr. Dean Ornish and used in a number of American hospitals has consistently shown that systematic use of diet, exercise, and meditation in combination can clear clogged arteries—promising large savings over the average $20,000–$50,000 cost of angioplasty and bypass surgery.[4]
- An eleven-year study used Blue Cross/Blue Shield data to analyze medical utilization patterns of individuals who practice Transcendental Meditation (TM: see chapter 24) as compared with normative data and matched control groups. The study found significant reductions in medical care utilization for program participants, including an overall 63 percent lower reate of medical expenditure compared to normative data, with an 80 percent reduction in hospital admission rate and a 55 percent reduction in the rate of out-patient doctor visits. Program participants over forty-five years old had 88 percent fewer hospital days than controls. Analysis by disease categories showed a 92 percent reduction in hospital admissions for immune, endocrine, and metabolic disorders; 92 percent

reduction for cardiovascular disease; 92 percent reduction for mental health and substance abuse; and 91 percent reduction for musculoskeletal disorders.[5]

Preventive strategies can create healthier citizens, cut health care costs, and alleviate untold anxiety, pain, and suffering.

Liming—Doing Nothing, Guilt-Free

*Every now and then go away, even briefly,
have a little relaxation, for when you come
back to your work your judgment will be
surer; since to remain constantly at work
will cause you to lose power.*

—LEONARDO DA VINCI

Liming is the Caribbean art of doing nothing, guilt-free, a revitalizing habit that's virtually unheard of in America. *Liming* can free you from the entanglements of convention and disengage the drive toward constant busyness. In its essence, all it takes is choosing one of your favorite healthy pleasures—such as telling jokes or flipping through an album of side-splitting cartoons. When you're starting to feel stressed or anxious, other *liming* suggestions include humming a heart-warming song, reading an upbeat aphorism or poem, putting on your sunglasses and listening to escape music while sipping iced tea, leaning back in your chair and looking out the window with your feet propped up on the desk and remembering your favorite vacation or funniest stories, or practicing a deeply relaxing meditation or visualization.

Liming, at its purest, is breaking away from the stress of time, of clock-watching. This kind of mental rest gives the brain a much-needed opportunity to sort out the load of information that has reached it during the past several hours. The truth is, as little as five or ten minutes of mental play-time during a work break can put you back in synch. Time off is not the same thing as time out. The basic idea with *liming* is to shift yourself out of the rat race—as completely and deeply as you can—for at least ten minutes, rediscovering the natural joy of human *being*.

UNPLUGGING

For many stressed men and women, the telephone—despite its obvious value—is the number one irritant in their busy lives. The crux of the problem appears to be too much communication and too little time alone. Unexpected phone calls during nonworking hours can interrupt reading, relaxing, and family time. The truth is that all of us need stress breaks. Somewhere during our hectic daily lives and on weekends, we each need opportunities to get away from phone interruptions.

But what if your job requires you to answer business calls twenty-four hours a day? Even in this case, it's essential to have some dependable way to rejuvenate your energies by leaving the battlefield—with an answering service, for example, or with the phone ringer turned off and the answering machine on during periods of unwinding. Do you really have to carry a portable phone with you on a dinner date? Do you need to have a phone in every room? Turning off the phone bell is a way to give yourself and loved ones some needed down time. You might deliberately let the phone ring without answering it at least once a day. Modern technology— pagers, websites, cell phones, faxes, and e-mail—is designed to empower you and set you free. In the information age, you must become a master of these technologies rather than allow them to control you. Unlike these techno-helpers, you were not designed to be on call twenty-four hours a day. That's why so many people suffer from automation anxiety and techno-stress.

INNER SCANNING

Many of us are so busy, so tense, that we fall out of touch with the subtle yet important sensory signals that arise from within the body. Without this awareness, we make it easy for stress to win; we fail to catch and neutralize negative pressures at their onset. An inner scan can help you detect tight muscles and relax them more easily. With practice, scanning can be used quickly—even instantly—to help you find and release tension.

Choose an environment that's free from distractions. Set aside about five minutes. Sit comfortably in a chair or lie on your back on a padded surface such as a carpet or bed. Spread your legs slightly, and relax your body. Close your eyes, and begin taking smooth deep breaths. Mentally scan a muscle area as you inhale. As you breathe out, imagine the tension releasing as that muscle area becomes more comfortably relaxed. After several breaths, shift your attention to another area. Systematically search your entire body: begin at the scalp and work down through the face, eyes, ears, jaw, tongue, neck, shoulders, upper arms, forearms, wrists, hands, fingers, chest, upper back, abdomen, lower back, pelvis, thighs, lower legs, ankles, feet, and toes.

For each body area you scan that is tight, mentally repeat, "Warmth and heaviness are flowing into my ____. Warmth and heaviness fill my ____ and it feels relaxed, comfortable, heavy, and warm. I feel my whole body relaxing ever more deeply as the heaviness and warmth fill my ____. I am letting go of all my tensions and worries. I feel peaceful and calm." Visualize the tension melting away—like an ice cube being heated by the sun and turning into a pool of water—as you exhale. Don't be alarmed if your mind wanders. Just bring your attention back and continue scanning.

Once you've finished, remain completely relaxed for a minute more. Notice the warm sense of ease in your body, especially in those places—perhaps the face, neck, jaw, shoulders, abdomen, or back—where you tend to hold tension. Can you feel your breath as it comes in and goes out? The slightest breeze on your cheeks or hands? The surface beneath your feet, legs, or back? Which arm or leg is more relaxed right now? The more senses you involve—sight, touch, sound, smell, and taste—the more you can restore inner balance and harmony.

UNLOCK YOUR BREATHING

Conscious breathing, the technique employed by both the yogi and the woman in labor, is extremely powerful. There is a wealth of data showing that changes in the rate and depth of breathing produce changes in the quality and kind of neurotransmitters.
—CANDACE PERT, PH.D., *MOLECULES OF EMOTION*

You can change your emotional state from worry and feeling threatened to self-confidence and a feeling of inner safety, by consciously altering your breathing. One of the most basic blocks to natural well-being is restricted breathing. Most people learn at a very young age to control feelings by holding their breath, and restricted breathing then becomes a habit in response to intense emotion. Surprisingly, most people halt their breathing for several seconds or more when they feel stressed. This reduces oxygen to the brain and pushes you toward feelings of anxiety, agitation, and panic. Situations that evoke fear, such as abusive parents or contentious siblings, can cause a child to grow up with chronic tension in the chest muscles out of fear of opening the heart. This results in poor posture and consistently holding one's breath.

Here is a simple exercise to gradually unblock your breathing. Sit comfortably, and loosen your clothes so that you can breathe easily with your abdomen. Now inhale deeply through the left nostril and hold for a count of four, then exhale through the right nostril to a count of four. Then inhale deeply through the right nostril, count to four, and exhale through the left to a count of four. Using your index finger and thumb to help you, continue this alternated breathing for three minutes, and let yourself enjoy it. The point is to breathe deeply, easily, and pleasurably. Notice the streaming energy with each inhalation as oxygen fills your lungs. You'll soon become very relaxed. If at some point during the day you feel tense, this exercise can bring relaxation in a matter of three to five minutes.

A remarkably effective on-the-spot technique for reducing stress and mild anxiety is one-breath relaxation. With practice, you can use one-breath relaxation whenever you start to feel jolted off balance by life's demands. First straighten your back and completely clear your mind. Now take in a deep breath of air. Don't force it; be *aware* of your breath coming in, *feel* the sensation—does the breath feel warm or cool? On inhalation, relax your shoulders, straighten your back, and let the air open your chest as you take a moment to be silent. As you deeply inhale, vividly imagine yourself drawing the breath into every fiber of your being, into every cell of your body, and imagine a bright light filling every corner of your mind. Hold the breath for a few extra moments, feeling it lift your spirit, and then, as you exhale, release every bit of darkness and tension from your thoughts and muscles.

Some people like to add a word or sound to help the mind focus as the breath goes in and out. Some individuals use *one* or *God* or *aum (om)*. *Hu* is an ancient sound for power. Many good words begin with *hu*: human, humor, hum, hub (the center), hug, huge, hue, humus (the good earth), humble, and, of course, hula. *Hu* is pronounced like the name Hugh. You can say it silently as you breathe in and again as you breathe out.

To make one-breath relaxation even more effective, you can link it to a specific and consistent hand position—perhaps pressing your thumb lightly against the tip of your index finger—as a memory cue. After a while, the touch alone can help elicit and deepen the immediate effects of one-breath relaxation.

One-breath relaxation is a simple technique, but it works. Many people feel the effects right away, and it can be used again and again throughout the day—as an easy way to stay calm when things around you are particularly hectic or tempers are short. A research study found that people who practiced daily breathing exercises were able to cut their levels of stress and tension in half.[1]

LEARNING TO LET GO

Trust thyself: every heart vibrates to that iron string.
—RALPH WALDO EMERSON

The simple act of safely letting go of control can become a wonderful means of stress reduction. What you resist persists; what you accept lightens. Just feel whatever you feel, and notice whatever you notice.

Select a quiet place and a comfortable position. Take the phone off the hook, or put a "Do Not Disturb" sign on the door. Loosen all constricting clothing. Give yourself full permission to let go. (Missing this simple step is one reason many relaxation plans don't succeed.) Let your eyelids close, and take a deep breath, filling your abdomen and entire chest. Repeat "Letting go" silently to yourself several times. Each time you exhale, imagine you're breathing all tension out from your body. As you exhale, repeat "Letting go" to yourself several more times. As your body relaxes and your emotions calm, unnecessary thoughts may parade through your mind. It's important not to fight or resist these thoughts—that only makes the distraction more powerful. Imagine that with each breath in, fresh, clean air is cleansing your mind of unneeded thoughts.

You cannot force yourself to relax—it doesn't work. Relaxation is basically a letting go process, so don't *try* to become relaxed. Gently, fully, place your attention on the sensation of tension without trying to fix it or change it. Just be with it. It's mindfulness and simple innocence that you're settling into. Bring into your consciousness positive words like "peace," "love," and "light" to assist you in letting go.

ONE-TOUCH RELAXATION

Here's one of the simplest and quickest ways to relax—anywhere, anytime. One-touch relaxation is achieved through gentle fingertip pressure on key muscles, which can trigger a cascade effect that quickly dissolves tension throughout the body.

Place your fingertips on your jaw joints just in front of your ears. Inhale for a few seconds, tightening your jaw muscles—bringing the upper and lower jaw together—which will feel like clenching your teeth. As you exhale, let the jaw muscles go totally lax, releasing all tension, letting the lower jaw drop, and relaxing your tongue. Notice the contrast between the sensations of tension and relaxation. Now repeat the exercise, but use only half the tightness in your jaw muscles. Hold for a few seconds, then release. Repeat with one-quarter of the original tension and then one-eighth—you'll find it much harder to discern these differences in tension.

You're using one touch to set the sensory cue for relaxation. You're specifically associating the sensation of your fingertips pressing on the jaw muscles with the highly desirable sensation of releasing tension. This process is triggered by a combination of your touch and the accompanying mental command to relax.

Again take a deep breath as you press and—using one touch with your fingertips against the jaw—relax these muscles with a full exhalation. (You should feel the jaw slackening.) Let your tongue relax and settle down into the base of your mouth, with its tip lightly touching your lower front teeth. Imagine yourself breathing out stress and putting aside your "shoulds," duties, and emotional burdens.

You can elicit a similar response by shrugging your shoulders, lifting them up toward your ears and then totally relaxing all of the muscles from your neck to your shoulders and across your chest and upper back, as you breathe away stiffness and release inner pressures. You can pick whatever other muscle areas of your body tend to stiffen up when stress mounts—such as the lower back or abdomen—and develop a similar quick-release technique for each of them. With practice you'll be able to reach up and use a single touch on your tense jaw, shoulders, or back to trigger an immediate wave of relaxation through that area, as if you're standing under a waterfall that washes away all tension and strain.

IMAGINE!

Imagination is more important than knowledge.

—ALBERT EINSTEIN

The word *imagination* is defined as "the formation of a mental image of something that is neither perceived as real nor present to the senses."[3] However, the images, thoughts, and feelings that flow from your imagination can have very real consequences upon your mental and physical health. When you are experiencing terrifying images and anxious thoughts, your brain cannot determine whether you are imagining a threat or actually experiencing one. In either case, the physiological consequences are the same.

Dr. Lennart Levi, noted stress researcher at the Karolinska Institute in Stockholm, Sweden, has shown that violent movies produce a substantial increase in adrenaline secretion, which can trigger fear and anxiety. In this light, it is not surprising that Dr. Bozzuto of the University of Connecticut has reported in the scientific literature a condition he calls *cinematic neurosis*. This disorder is characterized by such symptoms as insomnia, excitability, irritability, and hyperactivity, which develop in some people after viewing violent movies. Perhaps you have experienced a rapid heartbeat, hyperventilation, sweating, nervous tension, or tight muscles while seeing a horror movie or a *Die Hard* thriller. Just as experiences of cinematic terror are created by images and sounds on film, "inner movies" that regularly consist of frightening images or catastrophic thoughts can result in panic, anxiety, and neurosis.

Just as your imagination can produce anxiety, it can also create peaceful, healing experiences. The gift of imagination can be channeled to increase confidence, reduce fear, and ease sleep problems. Mental imagery can calm heart rate, respiration, brain-wave activity, and blood pressure. The way you focus your mind can even have beneficial effects on neurotransmitters, hormones, and the immune system. "The relations between emotion and immunity may prove to be another strong argument for a return toward whole-person medicine," stated an editorial in *Lancet*, one of Great Britain's leading medical journals. A 1997 study by C. Ashton *et al.* in the *Journal of Cardiovascular Surgery* demonstrated the beneficial effects of relaxation-visualization techniques for reducing anxiety in patients undergoing coronary artery bypass surgery.

With guided imagery, you choose to focus your mind on a specific visualization. While this valuable technique most often uses your "in-sight" (i.e., your inner sight), you can also enrich your experience with what you can feel, hear, smell, and taste. Include all of your senses to make guided imagery more vivid and effective. You may be someone who can visualize easily—perhaps thinking in pictures comes naturally to you. Some people's inner representations are more like a stream of verbal thoughts. Don't worry if seeing images in your mind's eye is not something you are used to. Even if your visualizations aren't clear, you will receive benefits. With practice, the power of your imagination can be strengthened to shape your health. Adding appropriate background music can make you an even better producer and director of your inner movie.

VISUALIZING AN ISLAND OF PEACE
Using your own or someone else's voice, you may wish to tape-record the visualization process described below. The

advantage of making a recording is that it allows you to listen, close your eyes, and focus fully on the imagery. Modify the visualization script to make the process more personal. To do the exercise, you will need about ten to fifteen minutes of relaxed, uninterrupted time. Put a "Do Not Disturb" sign on the door, and turn off the ringer on your telephone.

Take off your shoes, loosen your belt, and get as comfortable as possible. Sit in an easy chair or lie on a sofa, bed, or carpeted floor. Put a pillow under your head, and use a blanket to keep warm. Dim the lights, and perhaps put on some soothing background music. If you experience any nervousness or distress while practicing this guided imagery, just be easy until it passes. However, please know that you can stop the process and open your eyes at any time. If you like, you can seek professional assistance to help you gain more confidence in using the visualization exercises. Imagery skills usually take time to acquire.

Begin by using the relaxation and breathing exercises described earlier in this chapter to feel safe, comfortable, and calm. Now you are going to visualize your own island of peace, a place where you can go at any time to rejuvenate your mind, body, and spirit, to escape whenever you like from life's barrage of information and demands. Your own island of peace can put you in a relaxed vacation mode.

Breathe in slowly and gently, fully expanding your lower ribs as the air comes in and you arch your lower back. Breathe out smoothly as you imagine any worries and struggles floating away. Allow your mind to drift off to a secluded beach on your own island of peace. Rhythmic waves are gently splashing not far from your bare feet, and the water reflects the clear blue sky and the golden glimmer of the sun's rays. Feel the heat on your cheeks and shoulders and the soft dry sand beneath your feet. Take a step into the surf, and feel the cool wet sand between your toes. Feel the breeze picking up and drying you off. Notice how the breeze makes your skin feel cool and then hot again in the sun's pulsing warmth.

Now imagine yourself walking down the beach with a loose, carefree stride. You are deeply relaxed, drawing in deep breaths of fresh air, looking far down the shoreline to the distant horizon. You can see the white sand disappear into the emerald sea as a few small white clouds float in the timeless blue sky. You feel the awe and wonder of life pulsing in your heart. Take some time to relax and enjoy your island of peace.

Continue giving your imagination free rein. Just take it as it comes, neither anticipating nor resisting change. If you find yourself getting caught up in your daily demands, just gently ease off and bring yourself back to your island of peace. After about ten minutes, slowly open your eyes.

RELEASING FEAR AND LIGHTENING UP

Here is powerful guided imagery for releasing fear, anguish, or guilt. It can allow you to heal emotional conflicts that generate anxiety and to discover a source of inner peace. Light is the source of all life and warmth and therefore the source of all healing energy. Visualizing a healing light is used as an adjunct to conventional medical treatment, from healing wounds to cancer recovery. This healing imagery can help you lighten your emotional burdens. Follow the instructions below.

Unplug the phones, and put a "Do Not Disturb" sign on the door. Find a comfortable chair, or lie down, and give yourself a few minutes to relax and let go. Close your eyes and take five very slow, deep breaths, exhaling through your mouth. Begin to notice the soothing effect of settling down. Direct your attention to your toes, and feel them relax. Let your attention slowly glide up your body—feet, ankles, calves, knees, thighs, hips, abdomen, back, chest, neck, arms, face—and stop at each part to feel relaxation taking place.

Now imagine that you are floating in space or lying in a warm meadow. Create any mental image that you find peaceful, relaxing, and enjoyable. Let the world slip away, and drift naturally in your reveries. From this safe and relaxed place within you, perceive yourself without self-criticism. You can feel the release of letting down your guard. As you progress in your relaxation, you can feel the love and peace deep inside you.

When you are feeling relaxed and comfortable, picture the person(s) you feel you have hurt, as realistically as possible. Observe your feelings and thoughts as they occur. You may experience some tension in your chest, shoulders, or neck. Your breathing may become shallow or feel constricted. Without resisting the feelings and sensations as they arise, continue to focus your attention on the peaceful images you created during relaxation. Remember to breathe slowly and comfortably, letting go of any tension. Continue to relax, unwind, and feel more comfortable.

Imagine a white light surrounding you. Let it fill you with healing warmth and grace. Imagine this light focusing specifically on the area of your body in which you experience anxiety or remorse: your stomach, perhaps your heart, maybe your head. See your emotional pain surrounded by this goodness and light. Now imagine the light penetrating and dissolving the anxiety or guilt. The more the light saturates the guilt, fear, or hurt, the lighter you become. Imagine any remaining anguish entirely diffused in the light. As the darkness in a room is dispersed when you turn on the light, your self-punishment is no more. Be at peace in the goodness and light.

Use this visualization process daily for a time to help lighten and further dissolve your emotional burdens. Each time you do the exercise, take a few deep breaths and imagine a healing light sweeping over you. The light can be seen as emanating from any source comfortable to you—God, spirit, or love.

This inner light can assist in healing the pain and bitterness in your heart. Relax for five or ten minutes in this inner light. If you experience lingering pressure in your head or irritability after the exercise, be sure to take additional time to rest. Lie down, take some deep breaths, and let yourself unwind. You may practice this technique as much as needed until your heavy feelings lose their intensity and become lighter.

ANCHORING INNER SAFETY

An *anchor* is a single nervous-system cue that can elicit from memory sensations of feeling confident and being at your best. With a bit of practice, you can create a personal anchor that enables you to instantly shift your mind and elicit a surge of confidence and calmness under pressure.

In truth, countless anchors, or triggers, are affecting your behavior every day. For example, think of the immediate wave of emotions and memories that arises when you hear a favorite song. Or the forceful feelings you get from recalling one of your great (or worst) moments in a love relationship, parenting, or work. These anchors can be good or bad, strengthening or weakening, empowering or victimizing. The important fact is that they're everywhere. You can choose to either take greater charge of your life by forming anchors of inner safety and strength, tapping into a deep safe space within yourself, or make no effort at all and let your environment and the people around you dictate your emotional reactions.[4]

Here's a way to create a powerful personal anchor of inner safety. Sit in a comfortable, quiet place, and close your eyes. Direct your attention to your breathing, focusing on the air as it gently passes into and out of your nostrils and chest. Begin to feel the sensations of your body—air or clothing on your skin, the weight of your shoulders and arms, the texture and support of the surface you're sitting on, and so forth. Now draw your awareness to the center of your chest, to your beating heart. Whenever you notice your attention wandering, gently return it to the center of love and warmth in your chest.

Now vividly imagine yourself thinking, feeling, looking, sounding, and performing at your relaxed best in a specific past place and circumstance—a peak experience—when you felt safe, calm, and confident. Picture the safest moments of your life, as a child, as an adult, in the past year, or in the past month. Visualize yourself at your best, at a time when you were able to respond effortlessly no matter how intricate or demanding the challenge.

Recall your finest moment in great detail. Etch it into your awareness so that you can summon it in an instant whenever you choose or need to. Develop every aspect of this mental image of confidence, strength, and calmness. How deeply at ease are you? Do you feel a sense of adventure or discovery? What does it feel like to have this sense of mastery and balance? Are you indoors or out? In sunlight or shade? Rain or snow? What is the temperature? Do you notice air currents? What are you wearing, and how does it feel on your skin? What can you see in all directions? How do the muscles in your body feel? What is the rhythm of your breathing? What sounds are around you and off in the distance? Where is your mind focused? In what specific ways do you feel connected to nature and the universe around you?

At the peak moment of your image, make a unique sensory signal. Choose a touch, such as your thumb against the second knuckle of your index finger with a specific amount of pressure, and form a mental picture of yourself in a fluid state of confidence and relaxed alertness. These combined signals become your personal anchor.

Wait half an hour or so, and repeat the process. Later on, test your cue. Re-create the quiet, relaxed scene. Then, in slow motion, imagine a simple, specific phobia, but be certain to maintain the feeling that you are in a safe place while viewing the scene.

Research shows that with practice many fears can be overcome in this way. If you feel yourself becoming tense or anxious, make the barking dog less hostile or move it farther away from you in your mind until the sense of being safe and strong returns to you. Perceive the phobic scene, and then trigger your anchor. When your anchor is programmed into memory, it can be recalled, producing a quick surge of positive energy and inner calm.

With practice you can make the effect even stronger. If the anchor is well programmed into memory, for example, you can gain a few extra crucial moments of calm energy and self-control just by pressing your thumb and forefinger together. You are then less likely to freeze up or panic at the thought or the sight of a barking dog.

If your anchor doesn't seem to be effective at first, you probably haven't found vivid enough mental images or sharp enough sensory cues. Rehearse several more times. Again form the signal, increasing the richness and brilliance of the scene. How, exactly, does your best moment look, feel, sound, taste, and smell? Sense the lighting, colors, shapes, temperatures, textures, movements, physical sensations, and feelings. Be certain your sensory cues are unique, and see how they work for you. You'll be surprised how helpful such a simple tool, when practiced regularly, can be in mastering a phobia.

MUSIC AS MEDICINE

We are spectacular, splendid manifestations of life. We have language. We have affection. And finally, and perhaps best of all, we have music.
— LEWIS THOMAS, M.D.

Research has documented the powerful psychological effects that music can have on mood and emotions. The right song or melody can soothe frayed nerves. Listening to music you truly enjoy can give your nervous system a lulling massage. Hearing a tune or symphony that you love can dispel the "noise" of anxiety and create inner harmony. You can use music as a tool for stress reduction by itself or combine it with a visualization process, such as the previously described island of peace.

Alfred A. Tomatis, M.D., a French otolaryngologist, conducted research that demonstrated how music can recharge and retune the brain by dispelling tension and increasing enthusiasm. Music can lessen the level of stress hormones, blood pressure, respiratory rate, and stomach and intestinal contractions. Music is an inborn universal language system, which speaks to us so powerfully that it integrates memory and imagery with our innate healing capacity. A rhythmic beat can evoke tears, laughter, song, and dance. People are able to suspend their worries, release pent-up feelings, and become one with the composer or performer.

Find music that either nurtures, inspires, or relaxes you. You might choose Beethoven's Ninth Symphony, the Pachelbel Canon, an Enya album, birds chirping, or pouring rain. Whatever music or natural sounds you find soothing, just close your eyes and drift away. Vary your selections because after about twenty minutes the nervous system may become oversensitized to a specific tune and react to the tedium irritably.

Of course, music does more than just soothe or inspire. It can stimulate or enhance almost any activity, emotion, or mood—from crying to venting anger to dancing for pure joy. Lullabies, marches, dirges, and the Rolling Stones induce different feelings and states of arousal. Your natural self-healing program ought to include daily prescriptions of music. You can self-dose with music that charms, relaxes, or invigorates you.

"Music medicine" has become an active and important tool for healing anxiety and stress.

TRANSCENDENTAL MEDITATION

Within you there is a stillness and a sanctuary to which you can retreat at any time and be yourself.
——HERMANN HESSE, *SIDDHARTHA*

Meditation is attuning yourself to the music of your soul. It is traditionally considered a process that requires expert personal instruction for maximum benefit and understanding. If you have tried to learn a meditation technique from a book or magazine article and been disappointed with the results, you should not be surprised or discouraged. Your experience testifies to the age-old maxim that to learn to meditate properly you need a qualified teacher.

Among the various meditation techniques available, Transcendental Meditation (TM) is one of the most practical, easily learned, and effective programs. It's an ancient, time-tested technique whose benefits have been well established through modern scientific research. Qualified teachers are widely available to teach the technique and provide the necessary supportive follow-up, as well as advanced courses. While enrolling in the TM program is costly, you'll find that it is money well spent. You can attend an introductory lecture (no admission charge) at your local TM center. The address and telephone number can be found in your telephone directory.

Studies on the effects of meditation confirm that it can be of immense benefit to your health and total well-being. In meditation, you experience a state of very deep rest, marked by decreases in heart rate, breath rate, oxygen consumption, perspiration, muscle tension, blood pressure, and levels of stress hormones. You also achieve a state of heightened mental clarity and emotional ease, perhaps the result of increased coherence of brain-wave activity. One way to appreciate the significance of these effects is to contrast them with those produced by stress.

	STRESS	MEDITATION
Respiration rate	Up	Down
Heart rate	Up	Down
Oxygen consumption	Up	Down
Blood pressure	Up	Down
Muscle tension	Up	Down
Skin conductance (perspiration)	Up	Down
Stress hormone production (ACTH, cortisol)	Up	Down
Brain-wave coherence	Low	High

Numerous research studies have documented reduced anxiety and stress, measured both physiologically and psychologically, among those who practice the TM technique. One study found that the TM program was about twice as effective in reducing anxiety as any other meditation or relaxation procedure.[4] Other studies suggest that regular meditation may increase energy, heighten self-esteem, improve learning ability, reduce high blood pressure, and promote deeper sleep. Meditation elicits a unique state of the body, mind, and spirit that is the exact opposite of stress—a "stay and play" instead of a "fight or flight" response.

Research on the Transcendental Meditation program has consistently demonstrated both cross-sectional and longitudinal health benefits. A five-year sutdy of 2000 subjects has shown that people who practice TM have health care utilization more than 50 percent lower than matched control groups. The reductions were greatest in the oldest age group (averaging 67 percent lower) and in high-cost areas (the TM group needed 76 percent less surgery and suffered 87 percent less heart disease.)[5] A recent study on hypertension in elderly African-Americans found that Transcendental Meditation was twice as effective in reducing high blood pressure as progressive muscle relaxation and about equally as effective as medication, but without harmful side effects.[6] A further study found that Transcendental Meditation was more cost-effective in the treatment of hypertension than any of five classes of hypertensive drugs studied.[7] And a longitudinal study of 677 health insurance enrollees in Quebec showed that health care utilization declined between 5 percent and 7 percent per year after the subjects learned the Transcendental Meditation program.[8]

A meta-analysis of studies on reducing alcohol, nicotine, and drug consumption found that the Transcendental Meditation technique produced a significantly larger effect on stopping consumption than conventional treatment and prevention programs specifically designed to motivate people to quit.[9] Moreover, in contrast to the time course of conventional programs, whose initial success rates drop off precipitously in the first three months following completion of treatment (and continue to decline gradually thereafter), the time course for the Transcendental Meditation technique showed that abstinence patterns were maintained or increased up to two years later (the longest period studied).

25

Emotional Freedom

*The last of the human freedoms is to choose
one's attitude in any given set of circumstances, to choose one's own way.*
— VIKTOR FRANKL, M.D.

How much freedom of emotional response do you have?
Can other people easily intimidate you? Emotional freedom
is recognizing your power to respond and not just react; to
choose your experiences and behaviors. Discovering emotional freedom is not simple. Obviously, events over which
you have little or no control can happen in your life. Personal loss rightfully begets sadness and tears, just as great
success generates energy and joy. The point is, however,
that emotional responses need not be reactive, rigid, and
automatic.

Most anxiety is the result of predictable stimulus-
response patterns. Your spouse comes home tense; you take it
personally and get upset. Your lover gets angry; you feel
guilty or intimidated. You can, however, learn to be less reactive, even under trying circumstances. As herbs start to heal
your nervous system, you can choose to feel happy and loving
much of the time. Emotional freedom is neither self-deception

nor forcing a happy face when you feel nervous. No one receives 100-percent approval. Trying too hard to please will run you ragged and cause unnecessary anxiety. Pleasing or being pleased all the time is impossible.

PERSONAL RESPONSIBILITY— THE ABILITY TO RESPOND

A life of reaction is a life of slavery, intellectually and spiritually. One must fight for a life of action, not reaction.

—RITA MAE BROWN

Essential to achieving emotional freedom is learning to take personal responsibility. Blaming and complaining don't work. Chances are that when you're upset, you tell yourself, "I'm feeling tense because that person made a critical remark," or "I'm afraid because my spouse doesn't understand me," or "I'm annoyed because that person cut in front of me in line." The problem is that reflex comments like these place the blame for feeling anxious outside of yourself. When you blame someone or something else for the way you're feeling, you give that person or situation the power to control your emotional state. This perception forces you to wait until someone or something else changes before you can feel better, and these things are often beyond your control. Even if blaming gets someone close to you to change, they do so for the wrong reasons.

If, at the moment when you first feel yourself getting upset or anxious, you pause for a few seconds, without saying a word, and take full responsibility for how you feel and respond, it's easy to see the many choices you have and to realize that you can choose not to feel like a victim of cir-

cumstance. The next time you catch yourself blaming someone or something else for the way you feel, stop and ask
yourself whether it makes sense to put control over your
well-being in someone else's hands. Complaining is an ineffective way of getting what you want. By assuming that
someone else has control of your feelings, you remain caught
in an anxious rut.

People who benefit from psychotherapy, regardless of the
type of treatment they undergo, often report that they have
become emotionally "response-able,"—able to respond more
appropriately and express their feelings of fear, hurt, pain, loss,
and anger and the subtleties of love more effectively. Emotional
freedom allows you to diminish anxiety in fear-producing situations by becoming more outspoken, less inhibited, and better
able to express your needs. Your communication is committed to
a positive outcome and shaped by the following characteristics:

- Gets immediate attention through assertive but warm
  requests ("We've got to talk now, I'm frightened—"; "I'm
  upset and need to explain why—"; "I'm hurting, please
  give me your attention")
- Communicates hurt using *I* statements ("I feel fearful
  when you—"; "I feel let down, disappointed when you—";
  "I'd prefer if you would—")
- Communicates specific requests for change ("I get scared
  when you don't call me if you are going to be late"; "I'm
  hurt when you ignore me at a party"; "I'd like it very
  much if you introduced me to your friends because I get
  shy around new people")
- Leaves you open to other people's feelings and points of
  view ("I can see how you feel"; "I understand now my
  miscommunication"; "We'll need to watch out for—"; "I
  know you're trying, and I appreciate it"; "You're helping
  me feel more safe and secure")

Learning to recognize and express your emotions in a mature and honest fashion takes practice. Communication skills are just like athletic or musical skills—the more you practice, the more skillful you become.

PROBLEMS DON'T HAVE TO MAKE YOU MISERABLE

Nobody, as long as he moves about among the chaotic currents of life, is without trouble.

—CARL JUNG

To some, this idea may seem revolutionary, but your problems don't have to make you miserable. You can feel good about yourself and your life even when you have problems. You will always have your share of difficulties, in the midst of which you can choose to be satisfied, healthy, and loving.

Many people think that anxiety, worry, and tension are unavoidable as long as they're struggling with a problem. Beliefs such as "I have to solve my problems first" or "I have too many unsolvable problems" can become a justification for continued anxiety and misery. Such attitudes toward problem-solving can reinforce the unrealistic notion that you must become problem-free to become more relaxed and happy. This misguided belief is a nasty trap that not only prolongs distress but undermines your ability to solve problems.

A simple but important principle is that you think best when you feel best. The way to maximize your ability to solve a problem is to not let your happiness and well-being depend on it. Even in the midst of problems, give yourself permission to relax and enjoy yourself fully. Taking time to feel as good as possible is a wise choice to make.

A personal problem can be seen from two very different perspectives. Most of us start with a sense of frustration that we aren't living up to our own or someone else's picture of perfection. We berate ourselves with thoughts like "How could I be so stupid?" or "I just can't seem to do anything right." The attitude that a problem is a shameful deficiency stems from a basic perception that we are flawed. We secretly fear that we are defective and unworthy because of these shortcomings.

Many people punish themselves with internalized "shoulds"—rigid and demanding personal rules. The renowned psychiatrist Dr. Karen Horney first described "the tyranny of the should." If your "shoulds" have been weighing heavily on you, it's time to declare your independence. Ask yourself, "Who is making the rules in my life? My parents, society, or me?" Take an inventory of the "shoulds" that are causing you the most trouble. You might even write them down. Learn to substitute a softer "It would be nice if—" for your harsh, demanding "shoulds." For example, "I shouldn't have done that" instead becomes a lighter "It would be nice if I had made a different choice."

To heal anxiety, you may have to give up straining to be someone you are not, hiding the parts of yourself you fear are unacceptable, and worrying about what others think. You may have to forgive yourself for not being perfect and stop expecting superhuman feats from yourself. Indeed, you may have to accept yourself as you are instead of as you think you should be. The next time you engage in self-put-downs for not living up to some unrealistic standard, ask yourself, "Who am I trying to please? Whose approval am I desperately seeking?" It's time to set these punitive expectations aside and make your own reasonable preferences and standards.

WHAT YOU PLACE ATTENTION ON GROWS STRONGER

Whatever you direct your attention to increases its role in your thinking and action. This is an obvious basic principle that few people seem to appreciate. Instead of choosing to put their minds on constructive thoughts and useful actions, they exhaust themselves complaining about how they feel or why they can't be happy. Every time you indulge in complaining or pointless criticizing, you give whatever is upsetting you greater control over your life. It's like flypaper: the harder you try to shake it off, the more it sticks to you.

Only you should be able to decide what gets to dominate your experience. This is one of the fundamental rules of emotional well-being. If you allow yourself to be briefly but consistently conscious of constructive and supportive thoughts, your whole experience will expand in that direction. Emotional freedom lies in the ability to shift your attention, even slightly, in one direction or another.

This point may seem to be insignificant. In fact, it is the essence of personal freedom and an essential skill for mastering fear. If you allow your awareness to be consistently dominated—without inner argument or struggle—for a brief period of time by relaxed, confident thoughts or images, you can shift the direction and quality of your whole emotional experience. The father of modern psychology, William James, wrote that "The essence of genius is knowing what to overlook."

F.E.A.R.—FALSE EXPECTATIONS APPEARING REAL

There is nothing either good or bad but thinking makes it so.

—SHAKESPEARE

Psychologists have discovered a number of ways in which distorted thinking can magnify anxiety and stress. When you blame yourself for bad events but feel powerless to change them, feelings of distress rise sharply. This phenomenon is called *cognitive distortion*—automatic thinking that can lead to F.E.A.R. (false expectations appearing real). Do your thoughts and feelings serve you well? Do they work for or against you? Have fearful thoughts become *psychosclerotic*—rigid, automatic, and mechanical?

Fortunately, there are some rapid, well-proven ways to identify and then correct distorted, anxious thinking. These are some of the most common distorted thought patterns that contribute to needless anxiety:

- *Catastrophizing:* You exaggerate risks and problems, anticipating disaster or assuming the worst.
- *Guilty thinking:* Your self-talk is filled with "shoulds" and "shouldn'ts," "musts," and "oughts." When you break these rigid rules, you feel anxiety and frustration.
- *Disqualifying the positive:* You reject positive experiences on the grounds that they somehow "don't count" when compared with the endless list of problems at your job and in your life.
- *Either/or thinking:* There is no middle ground—things are either wonderful or terrible. Either you perform perfectly or you're an absolute failure.
- *Emotional reasoning:* You automatically assume that your feelings are facts and therefore must reflect the way

things really are. If you *feel* incompetent or inadequate, then you must *be* incompetent or inadequate.

- *Jumping to conclusions:* You quickly leap to negative interpretations of statements and situations, even though you may lack the facts to support such conclusions. This includes mind reading—without checking to find out the truth, you assume that you know precisely why other people think, feel, and act the way they do.
- *Blaming:* Your problems are either *never* your fault (other people and situations cause whatever goes wrong) or *always* your fault.

Distorted, fearful thinking is contagious—the habit spreads. When you consistently respond to events pessimistically, that negative style can amplify your feelings of helplessness, anxiety, and worry. Resist the natural tendency to accept distorted thoughts as true simply because they seem reasonable or "feel right." Begin paying closer attention to the way you explain unpleasant situations and outcomes to yourself. Identify negative, stressful thoughts, and examine them clearly and carefully, looking for supportive or contradictory evidence, alternative explanations, and more logical inferences. Derail the temptation to react with habitual anxiety and self-doubt.

OVERCOMING
SELF-DOUBT AND FEAR

Nothing in life is to be feared. It is only to be understood.
—MARIE CURIE

Self-doubt is at the core of much anxiety. Overcoming a lack of faith in yourself requires identifying your fears, which is the first step toward working through them. The following personal fears are common sources of self-doubt. See which of these barriers to self-confidence you recognize in yourself:

- *Fear of personal power:* When you take charge of your gifts and talents, you feel more confident, and your enthusiasm, energy, and motivation increase dramatically. Yet for some people this feeling of power is unfamiliar and even uncomfortable. When you have been living according to a dreary routine, owning your freedom can be frightening.

- *Fear of self-discovery:* Some people keep a tight lid on their inner life for fear of discovering something terrible about themselves. Such beliefs may be supported by parental or religious injunctions that self-esteem is conceit, pleasure is bad, and any enthusiasm is suspect. Many people cling tightly to the status quo to find protection from themselves.

- *Fear of losing control:* Some people suppress their desires the way a military dictator suppresses the populace, out of fear of revolt. They have needs and desires they want to explore, but they are afraid of losing control. At a party they want to let go and enjoy themselves more but fear appearing foolish or inviting gossip. They dream of being less rigid and less tightly controlled yet fear they might "run wild."

- *Fear of moving forward:* If you are prone to self-doubt, you may frantically search for reasons not to move forward. The more you resist making the best of the choices at hand, the more immobile and full of doubt you feel. For example, when you are afraid of committing yourself to a relationship, you can always find an eccentric habit, a minor shortcoming, or even an unattractive mole as reason to reject your partner.

- *Fear of making a "wrong" decision:* Some people remain stifled in a relationship or job they have long outgrown.

While a transition period is often filled with fear and uncertainty, nothing stands still in life. Not making up your mind is itself a decision. It promotes self-doubt, and you remain stuck.

• *Fear of letting go:* Some people go through life as if they're running the gauntlet, pushing themselves for every last bit of performance. They derive satisfaction from knowing they have lived through one ordeal and moved on to the next. Taking time to savor life is out of the question; they fear that slowing down means falling apart. Lurking underneath the compulsive hard work and achievement is a fear of emotional chaos or personal emptiness.

YOU ARE BIGGER THAN YOUR FEARS

You *are* bigger than your fears. Stop measuring yourself against a prefabricated ideal. When you were a child, it was appropriate to try to live up to the expectations of your parents and peer group. It is no longer appropriate to punish yourself for not living up to the expectations and images of others. Trust your desires and opinions by following your inclinations and instincts more often. Firmly tell your doubts, repeatedly if necessary, to stop or go away, and turn your attention to something more self-affirming. For example, list ten specific things about yourself in which you take pride. Include talents, determination, friendships, skills, and goodwill. Put this list on your bedroom nightstand, and review it before going to sleep and before getting out of bed each day.

Eliminate the words *wish, hope,* and *maybe.* Such words can erode your self-confidence by encouraging doubt, fear, and hesitation. For example, instead of saying, "I hope things get better," substitute "What I can do to find good work?" Do what you really love, and your life can become an adventure. Fear can be converted to excitement, a stimulus to break through your limitations. Rather than giving in to your fears, take reasonable risks in small but steady increments.

STOP TREATING YOURSELF AS FRAGILE

Argue for your limitations, and sure enough, they're yours.
—RICHARD BACH

With anxiety often comes a fear of falling apart if you make a significant change. This belief is a self-fulfilling prophecy that can keep you absolutely paralyzed. Albert Ellis, Ph.D., teaches, "One of the most harmful, irrational ideas of our culture is that danger, failure, or other stress is catastrophic."

The only way to stop thinking of yourself as fragile is to put your psychological strengths to the test. You will only realize how strong you are when you take specific steps toward change. It may not be easy, but you won't fall apart. Developing your psychological strength is just like developing a physical ability. The more you exercise, the stronger you become.

How can you make anxiety a stimulus and not a handicap to your personal growth? What skills and creative options can you pursue to transform this vulnerability into a source of strength? You have only a nagging sense of anxiety to lose and a growing feeling of power and satisfaction to gain. As painful as anxiety and stress can be, they can be a potent force for positive change, but only when we learn to perceive them as opportunities for new learning and growth.

There is much to be gained from cultivating an attitude of *healthy optimism,* which refers to positive expectations for what the future holds. As used here, the word *optimism* does not refer to the giddy optimism of pop psychology, mental pep-talk jingles, or Pollyanna but rather to flexible, real-life hopefulness. Although far from a panacea, optimism can make you more resilient when stressed.

FEELING IS HEALING

Our culture encourages us to be emotional illiterates, repressing our feelings or living at the mercy of emotional storms.
—DANIEL GOLEMAN, PH.D.

Fear and anxiety can come from a failure to identify more deeply what you're really feeling. Although expressing feelings may initially make you feel more vulnerable, it ultimately makes you feel safer and more connected to others. The feelings you resist persist; feelings that are shared can be healing. The next time you feel anxious, see if you can identify more specifically what you are feeling:

Odd	Abandoned	Fearful
Strange	Crushed	Intimidated
Persecuted	Agonized	Foolish
Petrified	Alone	Forgotten
Pressured	Angry	Frustrated
Sad	Blue	Hateful
Panicked	Affectionate	Afraid
Enraged	Apprehensive	Free
Rejected	Argumentative	Furious
Remorseful	Awed	Greedy

Resentful	Betrayed	Guilty
Restless	Bitter	Gullible
Jealous	Desirous	Flustered
Quarrelsome	Annoyed	Frightened
Scared	Bored	Helpless
Evil	Burdened	Homesick
Shocked	Challenged	Horrible
Sneaky	Cheated	Impatient
Sorrowful	Combative	Impressed
Sorry	Competitive	Inadequate
Resented	Awful	Grieving
Pitiful	Ambivalent	Frantic
Spiteful	Confused	Infatuated
Startled	Conspicuous	Infuriated
Stingy	Crazy	Insignificant
Stressed	Defeated	Isolated
Stunned	Despairing	Jumpy
Stupid	Destructive	Lazy
Suffering	Determined	Lecherous
Suppressed	Different	Left out
Surprised	Diminished	Lonely
Weak	Exhausted	Nutty
Mad	Disappointed	Longing
Tempted	Dishonest	Lustful
Distraught	Melancholy	Talkative
Tense	Disorganized	Explosive
Mistreated	Obnoxious	Vile
Tentative	Distracted	Mean
Dominated	Terrible	Threatened
Worried	Envious	Naughty
Tired	Exposed	Used
Neglected	Excited	Nervous
Terrified	Disturbed	Miserable
Obsessed	Bewildered	Hung over

If you communicate feelings (e.g., "I feel hurt by what happened," "I feel upset about what you just said," "I'm scared to be alone"), the stress of unexpressed feelings will often ease. Unaired feelings promote a sense of isolation; shared emotions help us connect heart-to-heart. Of course, depending on whom you're talking to, discretion must be balanced with openness.

JOURNALING

Some of the most effective and meaningful ways to reduce stress are to express fears, admit mistakes, and reveal secrets. Acknowledging your fears in writing can be an important step in healing. A significant emotional release can come from spending up to fifteen minutes a day writing in a private journal about things that are upsetting you. You need to give yourself permission to express the hurt, fear, anger, and loss connected with your anxiety. You need only a blank journal, a pen, a quiet place, and some uninterrupted time to write down your deepest feelings. The benefits of writing depend on spontaneously letting go and not censoring your emotions. Remember:

- Be honest, and don't overanalyze.
- Don't edit your thoughts or worry about looking good. Your feelings are enough in their raw form.
- Don't spend your time blaming or criticizing. These are also defenses against emotion. Simply express your fear, hurt, frustration, and pain.
- Don't try to defend yourself or to change anyone.

The suggested openers below can help you to express your anxiety, fears, and insecurities:

"I feel scared when—"
"I dread having to—"
"I am insecure about—"
"My worst fears are—"
"I feel trapped when—"
"I feel panicky about—"
"I feel rejected when—"
"I am embarrassed to admit—"
"I get anxious when—"
"I felt angry because—"
"I was hurt by—"
"I get frustrated when—"

Entrusting a troubling secret or painful feelings to a journal can bring relief.

WHEN IS PSYCHOTHERAPY NECESSARY?

So far I have emphasized how you can heal mild to moderate anxiety with herbal medicines or by committing to a program of natural self-healing. Nevertheless, there are situations where you can also benefit from therapy. Together with self-help, psychotherapy may be valuable when dealing with particularly troublesome issues.

There is nothing mysterious about psychotherapy, and therapists certainly cannot perform magic. They will not solve your problem but will help you discover how to solve it yourself. A psychotherapist is essentially a person who has specialized in helping others discover how to solve their emotional problems and learn interpersonal skills they did not develop while growing up. A therapist who is a psychiatrist can also prescribe medication if necessary.

Certainly most of life's difficulties or emotional crises do not require professional help. If anxiety is moderate to severe, however, psychotherapy with a mental health professional may be useful or necessary in the following instances:

- If herbal medicine and self-healing techniques are ineffective
- If you are caught in deep inner conflict
- If you don't feel good about yourself most of the time
- If you seek anxiety relief in a liquor bottle, illicit drugs, or binge eating
- If you feel perpetually out of control and under strain
- If you have personal problems that you haven't been able to resolve on your own after a sustained effort
- If you fear actually doing harm to yourself or someone else
- If you suffer from an obsessive-compulsive disorder
- If generalized anxiety, panic attacks, or post-traumatic stress disorder appear to be worsening
- If you're in a severe emotional crisis and the support of family and friends is insufficient
- If you suffer from disabling phobias
- If you are afraid that you may act on suicidal thoughts or rage
- If you are increasingly isolated emotionally or are socially withdrawn
- If you are suffering from a psychiatric disorder

COGNITIVE-BEHAVIORAL THERAPY

"Do you find yourself in the same unhappy situation again and again, wondering where you went wrong and why it happened again? It's not always just bad luck, it may be bad ideas," emphasizes Arnold A. Lazarus, Ph.D., the founder of multimodal behavior therapy. Effective self-help books can be used as homework to facilitate progress in therapy (see appendix A).

The major approach to anxiety disorders is cognitive-behavioral therapy, which employs proven, effective strategies for reversing them. Cognitive therapy identifies the distorted thoughts and perceptions that contribute to an individual's anxiety. The anxious person perceives life through a fearful prism. Cognitive therapy does not substitute rose-colored glasses but rather clear glass, which allows the world to be perceived accurately.

Cognitive-behavioral therapy uses clinically effective strategies for resolving inhibitions, desensitizing fears, and increasing assertiveness. In one technique, *role-playing*, the therapist models the new behavior (e.g., developing assertiveness by asking your boss for a raise), and you practice the demonstrated behavior until you feel comfortable with it. With a second technique, *systematic desensitization*, the therapist takes you through a step-by-step process to relieve specific phobias.

A remarkable study by UCLA researchers demonstrated that 18 patients suffering from obsessive-compulsive disorder (OCD), who were treated with cognitive-behavioral therapy, were able to change brain activity. The patients were given brain scans before and after practicing cognitive-behavioral therapy techniques. Results showed that 12 (two-thirds of the patients) had significantly reduced activity in the caudate nucleus, an area of the brain that has been shown to be overactive in OCD.

Patients with post-traumatic stress disorder, panic attacks, phobias, and depression can derive significant benefit from cognitive-behavioral therapy. It can also help with chronic fatigue syndrome. A study published in the March 1997 *American Journal of Psychiatry* showed that when patients with chronic fatigue syndrome received cognitive-behavioral therapy, 70 percent experienced substantial improvement in *physical* functioning, with a significant reduction in fatigue.

HOW TO CHOOSE A PSYCHOTHERAPIST

> *Come to the edge.*
> *No, we will fall.*
> *Come to the edge.*
> *No, we will fall.*
> *They came to the edge.*
> *He pushed them,*
> *and they flew.*
>
> —GUILLAUME APOLLINAIRE

Most people spend more time buying a car than searching for the right therapist. But research indicates that the empathetic ability of a therapist is as critical as theoretical knowledge in determining whether you will benefit from counseling. Therapeutic strategies and techniques can be very powerful when used by a therapist who is inherently helpful and genuine. Other characteristics to consider are authenticity, nonpossessive warmth, and a sense of humor.

The importance of choosing a psychotherapist carefully cannot be overemphasized. Seek referrals from your family physician, trusted friends, or national mental health associations (see Appendix D). Visit two to three licensed therapists with the intention of determining who would be most suitable. When making your final decision, consider the following questions:

- Is the therapist a licensed psychotherapist who is respected by the professional community and general public?
- Does the therapist have a pleasant disposition, a sense of humor, and appear to be functioning well personally?
- Do you feel safe, comfortable, and at ease with the therapist?
- Is the therapist honest, nondefensive, and empathetic?
- Is the therapist willing to explain his or her approach to your problem, including strategies, goals, and length of time for treatment?
- Is the therapist rigid in approach or flexible and open to your input?
- Does the therapist treat you as if you are foolish, flawed, or defective or treat you as an equal?
- Does the therapist listen silently, like a blank screen, or do you feel you are getting some sensible and generally helpful input?
- Does the therapist answer your questions and concerns directly rather than always asking what you think?
- Is the therapist willing to apologize when mistaken or inconsiderate?
- Is the therapist supportive of using herbs to heal anxiety?
- Does the therapist give appropriate feedback, or are you left with constant doubts about how the therapist perceives you?
- Does the therapist seem more like a consultant or a controller?
- Do the therapist's strategies and techniques show care and concern for you as well as for others?

- If you are interested, is the therapist willing to see your love partner or other significant people in your life?
- After the session, do you feel more hopeful and empowered, with higher self-esteem?

Therapists should be willing to explain their assessment of your case, their strategies, and treatment goals. It is also reasonable to ask for an estimate of how long treatment will last. Significant benefit can often be obtained in a small number of sessions.

Anxiety can be an opportunity for growth. It can serve as an important early warning signal that something within yourself needs attention. Instead of reacting with worry or frustration, ask yourself, "What can I learn from this situation?" and "How can I turn my apparent vulnerability into a source of greater strength, compassion, and well-being?"

Most healing takes place in a spiral, not a straight line; we tend to take two steps forward and one back. Instead of coming down on yourself each time your anxiety reappears or your growth is temporarily sidetracked, give yourself added support and guidance at these times. Rather than being self-critical, you can nurture and coach yourself through difficult challenges.

All growth is a combination of both insight and behavioral change. Insight without change can be frustrating. For growth, one must also take specific steps to break the self-defeating patterns of your anxiety. Saint Francis of Assisi taught, "Start by doing what's necessary, then what's possible, and suddenly you are doing the impossible."

To break free from the web of anxiety, you may have to give up a lot. You may have to give up feeling sorry for yourself, straining to be someone you are not, hiding the parts of yourself you fear are unacceptable, and worrying about what others might think. You may have to forgive yourself and others for not being perfect and stop expecting superhuman feats from others and yourself. You may have to learn to accept parts of yourself that you have resented your entire life. Indeed, you can grow to appreciate yourself exactly as you are and not as you wish you could be.

Healing anxiety is a gift you deserve for being courageous enough to admit that to be alive is to be vulnerable. Your peace of mind, your love and work relationships, and your moment-to-moment vitality may be at stake. Choosing between self-defeating anxiety and the full expression of your uniqueness is up to you. Healing anxiety can be a lifelong personal challenge but one that can bring you satisfaction, compassion, and growth.

26

Ending Worry, Sleeping Deeply

Take an inventory of your worries to see if they've accomplished anything. Has worrying about something ever altered the outcome? How many of the catastrophes that you've worried about actually occurred? As Mark Twain wrote, "Worry is like a rocking chair. It goes back and forth but gets you nowhere." For your worry habit to persist, you must invest energy in your worries by allowing each one to dominate your awareness. Instead of dwelling on your worries, you can choose to favor something positive, such as making plans or setting to work on a creative project.

Next time you worry about someone you care about, do something constructive to show your love instead. If your spouse is coming home late and you're worried, do something around the house that your spouse will appreciate. Bake a cake or set out some wine and music for a little romance when your spouse comes home. It doesn't matter what you do as long as it's something concrete to express your love rather than indulging in worry.

Face your fear of powerlessness. If you're worrying about some potential disaster, ask yourself, "What's the worst that can happen?" Get a clear picture in your mind of this calamity. Now ask yourself what you would do if it occurred. Don't suppress your feelings of fear. Instead of worrying, make concrete plans for action. This will transform your worry into constructive concern.

If you just can't shake anxiety about some potential disaster—for instance, the fear that a loved one has had a car accident while driving home late—ask yourself two questions: "What is the likelihood that it will occur?" and "Can my worry affect this potential disaster in any way?" Distinguishing between high-probability catastrophes and low-probability catastrophes is a useful technique for busting worry. You'll soon see the futility of your anxiety and can turn your attention to more productive, life-supporting activity.

Most worrying begins with a particular style of thinking called *What-if,* which intensifies a feeling of threat and anxiety. What-if thoughts are usually accompanied by images of catastrophe and misfortune. An excellent means of reducing worry is to turn your what-ifs into so-what-ifs. It also helps to follow this thought with a *well-then* response to further calm your alarm. For example, "What if I say something silly?" becomes "So what if I say something silly?" followed by, "Well then, I might feel awkward for a moment, but no one else will really care."

If a worry won't leave you alone, use a technique called *thought-stopping.* This makes use of your ability to control the thoughts that pass across the screen of your awareness. To stop a worry cold, take a few minutes to sit down in a comfortable place, close your eyes, and either silently or quietly tell the worry, "Go away" or "Get out of my head." Usually repression of feelings through willpower is not useful, but with the worry habit it can be helpful.

Recognize the wisdom of accepting life's uncertainties and confusion. There are many aspects of your life over which you have little or no control. So why get worried or anxious? It's wiser to treat these uncertainties like the weather. Accept them and go on to other things. Worry never accomplished anything!

FAILURE IS PART OF SUCCESS

Success is going from failure to failure without loss of enthusiasm.

—SIR WINSTON CHURCHILL

Failure and vulnerability are an inevitable part of being alive. Watching my one-year-old daughter, Shazara, take her first steps, I learned a powerful lesson: It's not how many times you fall but how many times you get back up. Each person learns to walk by first stumbling many times. You must be willing to risk failure before you become accomplished at anything. Risk of failure is a necessary part of success. Some people are anxious because they are persistently driven by a fear of failure. Yet the very best hitters only get three hits out of ten times at bat. To succeed, you must know how to fail.

Have faith in yourself—your ability to succeed at what you attempt and to get back up if you fail. The philosopher William James wrote, "It is only by risking our persons from one hour to the next that we live at all." Often faith in an uncertain result makes the result come true. The greatest rewards of living come when you step out of the bounds of your ordinary existence and extend yourself beyond what you believe are your limits.

Don't let yourself be crippled by worrying about failure. If you hold back and never depart from your routine because you fear failure, you're letting approval needs get the best of you. The worst part of failure becomes what others might think. This is the basis of all performance anxiety, whether on the tennis court, in bed, in the classroom—wherever someone may watch how well you do. The only way to end performance anxiety is to stop worrying about how you'll do and how you'll look doing it.

You're too important to put up with anxiety about the obstacles in your life. The best antidote for anxiety is action. Instead of bemoaning your problems or worrying about the long way to a major goal, take the first step. If your job is suffocating you, stop complaining and put together your résumé. Get any assistance you need to make certain it's the best résumé you can possibly write. If you're in a relationship that is faltering, gather up the courage to have a long talk about your future with your lover. Don't put it off until tomorrow. Do it today!

Action, even one small step, breaks the illusion that makes personal problems seem insurmountable. You can only solve your problems one step at a time. Taking the first step has the amazing effect of reducing anxiety about any problem to a manageable level.

Once and for all, eliminate your tendency to procrastinate as a means of avoiding failure. First, make a list every morning of everything you have to do that day. Divide the list into areas: telephone calls, letters, housework, reading, writing, appointments, and so on. Make your list early in the morning so that it becomes a habit. Throughout the day, consult your list and cross off what you accomplish. Whatever remains at the end of the day becomes part of the next day's list. If an important item remains for several days, tag it and allot a special time of day to do it. This simple technique can help you end procrastination forever.

Don't be ashamed to ask friends for support when you consider a major change. You may have legitimate concerns about leaving your job, going back to school, moving to another city, or doing whatever seems necessary to create the life you really want. You may get very conservative advice from some people: "Don't take risks," "Don't rock the boat," "A boring job is better than no job at all." But you're also likely to get encouragement and help. People will respond to your courage. Doors will open. Try it. You'll be surprised how helpful people can be when you ask.

Decide to forego the crutch of old labels you've pinned on yourself to make excuses for remaining the way you are. You may say that you feel good about yourself, but your behavior may speak otherwise. Which of these forms of low self-worth apply to you?

- Feeling embarrassed about your abilities ("It wasn't skill, just luck." "Today was just a good day.")
- Giving credit to others when you really deserve it ("Martha did all the work, I just drew up the plan." You write a report and let your superior put his or her name on it.)
- Failing to stand up for what you believe (You criticize the President's policy; someone counters with a barrage of statistics; you back down.)
- Passing up an opportunity for fun because you feel you don't deserve it (Friends invite you to the beach/movies/park, but you stay home and work even though you need a few hours of relaxation.)
- Saying yes when you want to say no, in order to be a "good guy/gal" (A friend asks you to do an errand and you agree even though it's really not convenient, and you feel angry about it.)

Do you indulge in any of these self-negating acts? In what ways are you your own worst critic? What specific thoughts and behaviors reveal hidden feelings of inadequacy?

How do you put yourself down or fail to take the credit you deserve? Look for clues to your inner deforming mirrors and how you may be inadvertently training others to see and treat you. As Eleanor Roosevelt recognized, "No one can make you feel inferior without your consent." You have the power to create the life you want.

LAUGH!

Laughter is inner jogging.

—NORMAN COUSINS

Enlightenment may be lightening up; making your "heavies" lighter. You might try turning your worry into an opportunity for healthy laughter. Try setting aside ten minutes a day to do all your worrying. If you catch yourself worrying at another time, just tell yourself to wait until the designated time. Try this once or twice, and your worry period will soon become a laugh session as you realize how ridiculous it is to worry.

People who know how to have fun are generally better able to bounce back from stress. Humor has very little to do with telling jokes. It's about chuckling at the absurdities, hassles, heartaches, and hard times of everyday life and taking yourself more lightly. Striving for success is just another game that's not to be taken too seriously. No matter how talented and hardworking you may be, you can never win at every challenge. A sense of humor is essential to combating frenzy and the feeling that you're on a never-ending treadmill. The ultimate sign of success may be the ability to laugh and enjoy the simple pleasures of daily living.

Humorous thoughts and mirthful laughter work wonders by initially arousing and distracting the mind and then leaving us feeling more relaxed. Scientists theorize that laughter stimulates the production of the brain's endorphins, which are related to the easing of pain and feelings of joy. Cultivate cosmic humor. Spontaneous mirth is something you "allow" to happen naturally through a sense of relaxation and fun. Start looking for more of the ridiculous, incongruous events that go on around you all the time. Make up short stories about the funniest things you see or hear, and use them to spice up family and business discussions.

Laugh more. William F. Fry, Jr., M.D., Associate Professor Emeritus in the Department of Psychiatry at the Stanford University School of Medicine, suggests that laughing as much as a hundred times day is a healthful goal that's also fun. Start a humor library. What makes you laugh? Whether it's cartoons, letters from friends, posters, old or new comedy movies, joke encyclopedias, or humorous stories (in books or on audio tapes for listening while you work or drive), expand your collection. Pay attention to whatever tickles your funny bone—and make it a point to surround yourself with it.

DEEP, REFRESHING SLEEP

A well-spent day brings happy sleep.
—LEONARDO DA VINCI

Ironically, the greatest nightmare for chronic worriers is lying awake tossing and turning with their minds ceaselessly racing. Perhaps they finally get an hour or two of fitful, troubled rest, but upon awakening they find they are exhausted and frightened about keeping up the next day.

Sleep is meant to be a natural and deeply refreshing experience. It depends first and foremost on knowing how to unwind and let go. Sleep research has documented that a brief period of moderate exercise three to four hours before bedtime, such as a fifteen-minute walk after dinner, can significantly deepen sleep. Here's why: physical inactivity ranks among the prime causes of insomnia. Studies link physical fitness with improved sleep quality.

Sedative herbs such as valerian are excellent sleep aids. A warm herbal bath a few hours before bedtime can also be beneficial because of the sedative effects of the herb and because it increases body temperature. Your temperature will drop as you get ready for bed, a natural trigger to deep sleep. Researchers have found the use of lavender oil in aromatherapy can relieve insomnia and promote more restful sleep (see pages 130–131.

CREATE A TIMELESS BEDROOM

Man must not allow the clock and the calendar to blind him to the fact that each moment of his life is a miracle and a mystery.

—H. G. WELLS

Another good idea is to make your bedroom a time-free space. If you must set an alarm clock, place it where it can be heard but not seen. If you suffer from insomnia, it's best to keep time pressures out of your sleep environment. If you want the best possible rest, make it a rule to preserve your bedroom as a comfortable, relaxing haven and a place for a warm, intimate relationship. Nothing else. Keep heated discussions, intense brainstorming, computer work, and monthly budgets out of your bedroom.

Just as important, arrange for a gentle awakening. Leaping up to shut off an alarm clock is a jolt to your entire being, triggering a racing heartbeat, muscle tension, stressful "emergency" symptoms, and a raw emotional tone that can last all morning. A clock radio tuned to music you enjoy at a volume just loud enough to awaken you is a less stressful alternative to a traditional alarm. If possible, wake up a little earlier than you need to so that you can lie in bed, blink your eyes, move your arms and legs, and allow your body to awaken gradually. How you spend these waking minutes can have a great—and sometimes profound—influence on your peace of mind all day long.

FALLING CALMLY ASLEEP

People who are the most stressed and anxious often hold on to excessive muscle tension all night long. The result is that they end up feeling tired in the morning and more stressed throughout the day. Here's a method for calming down before you drift off to sleep.

First take several deep, pleasant breaths, and then concentrate on tightening and then relaxing the muscles in your face, jaw, neck, and tongue. Extend this tense-and-release process across your chest and shoulders, down your back and abdomen, and out to your fingertips and toes. You can also add soothing music, bedtime prayers, or positive affirmations for putting yourself at peace.

To enhance a pleasant drift into slumber—especially if you happen to find yourself feeling anxious about sleep—take a few minutes to breathe deeply and recall your fondest memories of soothing, wonderful sleep, perhaps from your childhood years or a restful vacation. If you feel a twinge of worry about falling asleep, you can avoid this by recalling bright, pleasant images and feelings of deep sleep, using these as a powerful anchor to ease the fear of insomnia.

There is an important link between what you eat and the

quality of your nightly rest. Don't go to bed hungry. If you eat an early supper and then skip a midevening snack, you can end up with a drop in blood sugar in the middle of the night that can awaken you from sleep. What are some good light nighttime snacks? Several low-fat cookies and a glass of milk, some air-popped or very low-fat microwave popcorn, a serving of fresh fruit and low-fat yogurt or cottage cheese, or some other high-carbohydrate, high-protein favorite. Foods such as these may help deepen your sleep by increasing brain neurotransmitters that promote a calm state of mind and relaxed emotions.

It is also a good idea to avoid coffee, tea, and other caffeinated beverages within four to five hours of bedtime. If you choose to drink alcohol in the evening, do it early—generally not less than three to four hours before bedtime. The reason is that although alcohol makes some people drowsy, it actually distorts the normal brain-wave pattern of sleep and prompts more frequent awakenings, sometimes causing difficulty in getting back to sleep. Please see chapter 14 for herbal prescriptions if insomnia becomes persistent.

27

Are You
Anxious or Angry?

We boil at different degrees.
    —RALPH WALDO EMERSON

Anger can be frightening. Some people find this basic, natural feeling so threatening that they reflexively block it out of awareness: "What, me angry? Never." The energy of anger doesn't go away, however; for many it changes instead into anxiety. The suppressed anger stemming from an unhappy marriage or a business difficulty can easily lead to anxiety.

The intimate relationship between anxiety and anger is best understood by examining the underlying physiology that these emotions share. As described in Part 1, when you feel threatened the first stage of the stress response immediately kicks in. This alarm stage is called the "fight or flight" reaction because it triggers a massive mobilization of energy for either fight (anger) or flight (anxiety).

When human beings had to survive in the jungle, this response could be lifesaving. If you came across a saber-toothed tiger, you had to mobilize quickly to fight for your life or swiftly flee. A modern person, however, is not too often confronted with a crisis that calls for either physical violence or escape from threat of harm. A man caught in a traffic jam is not making an appropriate adaptive response if he steps out of his car to fight, nor would a woman receiving an unfavorable evaluation from her boss be responding appropriately if she decided to take flight.

Given enough stress, hurt, or frustration, the human psyche responds with anger or anxiety as adrenaline pours into the bloodstream. You can't turn this response off; you've got to do something with it. If you fight it and lose control, it comes out in a destructive display of anger. If you block it because you find it frightening, it goes underground like a smoldering fire, resulting in chronic anxiety. The healthier choice is to accept the anger, let yourself feel it, then collect yourself and use the energy to deal effectively with what is troubling you.

When you get angry, you feel a surge of energy, your blood pressure increases, your muscles tense, and you may feel warm. You're likely to have destructive thoughts such as "I'd like to wring his neck!" or "I'd like to show her up for what she is!" Again, many people are uncomfortable with these powerful feelings. "I get nervous when I get angry," said one of my clients. "It makes me feel guilty," said another. These feelings lead to an internal struggle that inhibits the natural experience of anger and makes it more difficult to cope.

MAKING ANGER WORK FOR YOU

Stop for a moment and look objectively at the sensations of anger. What's wrong with feeling a surge of energy or a muscle tensing or a wave of warmth or a violent thought passing through the mind? These components of anger are neither good nor bad in themselves. They just are. Whether anger becomes destructive or constructive depends on how you channel the energies that anger releases in you. To control your anger, you must allow yourself to feel it. Paradoxically, the more you experience the power in your chest, the rising energy in your body, and the heightened alertness of your mind, the more control you have over your anger, and the less grip it has on you.

Sometimes it's useful to think of anger as a chemical reaction. When you apply heat to a piece of wood, carbon compounds react with oxygen, and the wood bursts into flame. Given enough heat and oxygen supply, the fire is inevitable. It's the same with anger.

Anger becomes positive when you shape your expression of it with these characteristics:

- *Warmth:* You release your feelings honestly and openly with strong words to let the other person know that you've been hurt.
- *A clear goal:* You want the person who hurt you to acknowledge your hurt and to agree on how you can avoid future misunderstandings.
- *Release:* It allows you to feel better, forgive, and forget. You completely release the tension that accompanied your anger so that you can see the relationship in a new light and be magnanimous about forgiveness.
- *Brevity:* You get your anger out in five or ten minutes by expressing it as directly and honestly as you can. This doesn't mean you'll move to understanding and forgiveness so quickly. The angry outburst may open doors to many issues that need examination. Their discussion may take time, but the hostility will be lessened quickly and the atmosphere become conducive to reconciliation.

CONSTRUCTIVE VS.
DESTRUCTIVE ANGER

There are two ways to get angry, and they differ in intent, quality, and outcome. You can explode because you want to pay someone back for the hurt he or she caused you. Whether you scream in rage or walk out in cold silence, the goal is the same: to punish the other person for an offense. Or you can use heated words and gestures to communicate your hurt and explain how you want the relationship to change. You may yell or curse, but you don't back down or walk out until you get your point across.

In the first case, your anger adds hostility, creates additional bitterness, and freezes the relationship around an event of the past. In the second case, your anger releases tension, facilitates an emotional breakthrough, and helps the relationship evolve to a new level of mutual respect, understanding, and appreciation. In the end, anger that punishes is destructive, whereas anger that communicates effectively is constructive.

When anger becomes infected with the desire to punish, it becomes twisted. Its effects on you and others are wholly negative. What can destructive anger do? A number of things:

- Weaken self-esteem and create a feeling of impotence because it exposes lack of self-control
- Mask your real feelings of hurt with cold indifference or a furious assault
- Inhibit communication and leave you feeling tense or bitter
- Create emotional distance, destroy relationships, and increase feelings of isolation
- Defeat its own purpose by making other people turn

away from you while compounding your own tension and
frustration
- Lead to ulcers, high blood pressure, and headaches when
you get locked into a defensive and chronically angry pose
- Accumulate over time and contribute to a general hostility and distrust that seep out in nasty bits and pieces

Anger becomes constructive when its specific characteristics contribute to healing the underlying emotional injury.
Constructive anger:

- Empowers you to stand up for yourself and stop putting
up with pain
- Helps you communicate your hurt so that you're free to
say, "I feel let down, betrayed, disappointed, and pushed
around."
- Enables you to break through a fixed and destructive pattern in a relationship
- Aims for mutual understanding so that the relationship
can be restored on a new footing where your feelings are
given more weight
- Expresses the stated purpose of changing the relationship in specific ways that will help avoid future hurts and
misunderstandings
- Prepares the emotional ground for forgiveness and forgetting once the relationship begins to shift to its new footing

RESCRIPT AND REHEARSE

Relax for a few moments. Take a deep breath, and recall a
recent minor conflict that turned into an angry exchange or
an argument, one that didn't end up as well as you would

have hoped. For example, possibly someone lit up a cigarette in a no-smoking area or cut in front of you in line, and when you spoke up, they launched into an angry war of words. The situation can be any kind of verbal assault but one where, at least at first, there was no physical violence.

Relive the experience in your imagination. Exactly what did it look like, sound like, feel like? Did you pause and remain calm? Or did you react right away? What were the facial expressions and voice tones like? What was the posture like? What specific words, gestures, or sounds seemed to make things better—or worse? Did any word or action *almost* turn things around and resolve the conflict? Were you or the other person, or both, trying to listen or to be "right"?

Now rewrite the script. Review the conflict in your mind as if it were happening right now. At the first moment you feel the clash beginning, trigger a split-second pause. Perceive more deeply this time, heightening your sensitivity to whatever the other person may be struggling with. In a friendly but assertive manner, say something like, "My intention is not to hassle you. I thought perhaps you had missed seeing the no-smoking sign." The point here is to try to give the other person the benefit of the doubt and a face-saving, argument-deterring opportunity.

MENTAL SHIELDING

One scientifically validated mental shielding technique is based on imagining a point of light in front of you, then stretching that point of light into a window of light. You use the light to mentally construct an instant titanium-like shield, a curtain of light, a screen, or a wall. You may want to wrap the shield or light all around you in a circle or protective sphere. Use whatever image is most comfortable for you.

With practice, you can focus your thoughts to give the shield protective qualities so that nothing angry, critical, or manipulative can pass through it. You can still see through this shield as an observer, and the protective barrier allows positive thoughts and feelings through.

In mental rehearsal, you remain relaxed and alert as you imagine a troublesome person in front of you making an accusation or threatening comment. You envision yourself observing the comment being hurled toward you and see it strike the shield, disintegrating or being deflected, then passing harmlessly by. You realize that the anger attached to the words does not have to affect you, and thus you experience being protected. This mental shielding technique is particularly valuable in light of evidence that when facing criticism and rudeness from others, it is often best to remain as alert, detached, and uninvolved as possible in order to remain safe.

The truth is that by brushing off insults and degrading words, you are not merely pretending. What you take as important or unimportant can literally help construct the reality of what follows. Perceiving an ugly comment as small and distant helps you keep the attack itself small and distant. You subsequently gain considerable power in controlling the meaning of your experiences. Likewise, no slight is so small, no rude word so minor or petty that it cannot be made huge and destructive by getting anxious or upset about it.

COMMON COMMUNICATION TRAPS

Many arguments have little to do with the issues or ideas being discussed. For instance, you and a loved one may quarrel over finances, the children, politics, home remodeling, or even your reactions to a recent movie. The anger and heated words are often less about the issue and more about the frustration that ensues from a failure to listen to each other's feelings and acknowledge each other's point of view. Ten maladaptive communication habits cause most of the problems.[1] I call these habits *anxiety-anger traps* because couples fall into them time and again. Look at the descriptions below, and see if you or your love partner are stuck in any of them.

ANXIETY-ANGER TRAP 1:"I'M RIGHT; YOU'RE WRONG."

Human beings can be incredibly self-righteous. Anxiety causes us to become rigid and defensive. In an argument, it is easy to recognize how right you are and how wrong the other person is. Neither side wants to give in, and both sides feel misunderstood. There is always a group of like-minded friends and relatives who unequivocally support how right you are and how obviously wrong your lover is.

When both lovers are defending "I'm right; you're wrong" positions, a simple discussion of a specific issue often evolves into a struggle of wills. You may think you're arguing the merits of an issue, but you wind up responding emotionally as if you're fighting for the survival of your own self-worth. Families are notorious in this regard. How often have you heard a simple discussion at the dinner table build to a heated argument, making everyone feel uncomfortable?

The "I'm right" syndrome can make it difficult if not impossible to accept valuable feedback from your lover. If your lover criticizes one of your cherished beliefs, you may feel so put down that you resist whatever he or she says, to the point of adamant defiance. Even if that criticism should invite little argument, such as a suggestion that you stop smoking, some people caught in the "I'm right" trap interpret it as an attack on their emotional survival. Well-intentioned criticism is vital to a healthy relationship, and overcoming the "I'm right" trap is crucial to allowing such healthy communication between lovers.

If you stop reactively insisting how right you are and try instead to listen receptively, you'll allow your love partner to be right as well. A key to nurturing every love relationship is to set aside your own self-righteousness and both acknowledge and value your lover's opposite point of view. Remember that reasonable people disagree about important matters all the time without becoming emotionally inflamed. If a simple discussion leads to a quarrel with your lover, the "I'm right" anxiety-anger trap is probably the cause. If you recall that when it comes to sharing feelings, no one is wrong, you and your partner will become less anxious about having emotional differences.

ANXIETY-ANGER TRAP 2: WIN/LOSE

Trying to "win" when you and your lover disagree is a futile endeavor. The urge to win is associated with the need to be one up and force your love partner to be one down. Such anxious competition inevitably leads to both lovers losing. Even if you "win," your lover feels resistant, defiant, and resentful for being turned into the loser, and you will soon pay for it in diminished affection or the next round of quarreling. A variation of this anxiety-anger trap is to fight over who is being "fair," and it is this petty, self-defeating bickering that leads to both lovers feeling cheated because neither gets what he or she really wants.

In any dispute with your lover, you must aim for a resolution in which you both win, you both are right, and you both get your wishes and needs fulfilled. While this resolution cannot always happen in business, it can happen very often in a healthy love relationship. Disagreements between lovers have to do with priorities, recollections, choices, judgments, values, opinions, and other purely subjective perspectives. Consequently, there is usually no absolute standard for measuring who wins or what is fair.

To find creative solutions to disputes with your lover, you need to begin by accepting each other's point of view as valid. For example, your husband shouts, "You should do more of the dirty work around the house; I slave to earn us a living." Trying to convince him that his feelings of working so hard are inaccurate or that you already do most of the "dirty work" will raise both his and your anxiety. Striving for a win-win solution means assuming that if you were in your love partner's shoes, you might feel exactly the same way. From that perspective, the effective response might be, "I understand how hard you've been working. I work awfully hard too, and I want to make things better for us. Let's discuss how we can make some positive changes."

That doesn't mean that you must bow down three times and meekly scrub the kitchen floor or iron the laundry. Rather, you communicate respect for your lover's feelings, and then together you examine practical solutions that serve you both. The more you can truly empathize with your lover while maintaining your own dignity and self-worth, the more your lover is likely to move from a rigid position and empathize with your fears, concerns, and worries.

ANXIETY-ANGER TRAP 3: DOUBLE BIND

A communication is called a *double bind* when it contains two contradictory messages. For example, your lover says, "Come here, darling," with hostility and venom in her voice. Do you come over or don't you? You feel ambivalent because you are getting a double bind message. Here is another example: He says, "Why do you have to do everything I tell you?" In this situation, what is the love partner to do? By complying with his demand, she is doing as he tells her, but by ignoring it, her behavior continues to irritate him. Another double bind is to demand behavior that can only be spontaneous: "Show me how much you love me," or "I want you to respect me more."

Even if you cooperate with these messages, you will do so with resistance as opposed to genuine love and respect. Double bind messages almost always leave you feeling anxious and dissatisfied.

The solution to the double bind message is to be straightforward. Beware of putting your lover in such a trap, and if your lover trips you up with a double bind, don't try to figure out what he or she really wants. Ask instead. Often the real problem is wholly unrelated to the initial confusing message.

ANXIETY-ANGER TRAP 4: EITHER/OR THINKING

Anxiety breeds inflexibility. Many people assume there is only one right answer to every question. In relationships, there is almost always more than one right answer, and the truth usually lies somewhere between two extremes. Nevertheless, many couples create hours of needless quarreling by taking the stubborn position that statements are either right or wrong.

Consider a typical domestic battle between lovers who think in all-or-none terms:

WIFE: You're always hassling me, always putting me down, and always finding fault with the way I raise the children and spend the money. I can never do anything right as far as you're concerned.

HUSBAND: That's not true; I never do that.

WIFE: Yes, it is.

HUSBAND: No, it's not.

WIFE: See, there you go again; disagreeing with me.

HUSBAND: I'm not disagreeing with you.

WIFE: Oh, yes you are.

HUSBAND: No, I'm not.

WIFE: So then, you admit that you always find fault with me!

This anxiety-anger trap can grow beyond what either

lover may have initially intended and can result in serious problems. All too many marital clashes hinge upon either/or thinking. Couples adopt opposite positions on money, sex, relatives, personal habits, the right way to discipline children, and so on. The result is a never-ending power struggle.

The antidote is to recognize that when it comes to beliefs and perceptions, there are multiple right answers. Compromise should be highly valued; it is not a sacrifice of some high moral position. The more you incorporate words such as *sometimes* or *often* and avoid terms such as *never* or *always*, the more you will avoid anxious bickering.

ANXIETY-ANGER TRAP 5: ASSUMPTIONS

Anxiety often leads to making assumptions. A common trap is assuming that you know better than your lover what he or she is really feeling and thinking. It is not unreasonable for you to perceive your lover's behavior differently than your lover does. It is unreasonable, and a breach of trust, for you to deny your lover's report of his or her feelings, thoughts, and experience. Assuming you know better than your lover what is best for him or her demonstrates a lack of respect and sensitivity. It also leads to accumulating resentments and a potentially serious crisis when one lover finally has enough of being pushed around.

Misuse of the word *we* is the classic expression of this anxiety-anger trap. The dominant figure in a couple (usually the male) may often say things like "We feel that—," "We disagree with—," or "We would like to—" when all that is really being said is "I feel that—," "I disagree with—," or "I would like to—." The more submissive and compliant love partner is not even asked for his or her beliefs, opinions, or point of view. Such behavior inevitably results in diminished self-esteem and a hidden resentment. If you assume too many *we's*, someday your lover will rebel. The solution to this anxiety-anger trap is very simple. Ask your mate how he or she feels, and accept the response as true. Also, do not speak for your love partner unless you've asked his or her opinion first.

ANXIETY-ANGER TRAP 6: DISAPPROVAL, JUDGMENTS

Excessive need for approval is a major factor contributing to unnecessary anxiety. People with this need tend to avoid criticism at all costs and invest other people's opinions and judgments with unreasonable value: "What will the neighbors/your mother/your lover think?"

Trying to please everyone all of the time is impossible. Some people, and that will occasionally include your mate, are bound to dislike something you say or do no matter how hard you try to please them. You and your lover may respect each other very much, but each of you is going to have some traits or behaviors of which the other disapproves. Rather than feeling anxious, hurt, or angry when you are faced with such disapproval, it's best to recognize that some criticism is healthy in any love relationship. The more you accept it as feedback rather than rejecting it, the more you will create a sense of self-approval.

To avoid this trap, be careful to distinguish between facts and judgments. For example, "I work as a full-time housewife" is a fact. "I am *only* a housewife" is a fear-based judgment. The judgment may proceed further as follows: "I should have gone to college and taken up a profession. My failure to do so is a shameful disgrace. My spouse looks down on me, and so does everyone else." Thus people apologize for their backgrounds, jobs, or homes and go through life feeling ashamed. When you live in fear of judgments, you constantly punish yourself and naturally feel anxious and angry measuring yourself against other people's standards.

Every effort should be made to become less judgmental toward yourself and others. This is especially critical in a love relationship because you train your lover how to view and treat you. If you believe you are unworthy because you are only a housewife, then it's possible that your love partner will reflect this image at you, leaving you feeling rejected and insecure. If, however, you feel great about being a housewife, mother, and domestic engineer and recognize your work as one of the most important and vital professions in the world, then you will train other people to see you and what you do with great dignity.

ANXIETY-ANGER TRAP 7: STRESS

Under stress, there is a tendency to revert to old habits. With increasing pressures and demands outside the relationship, it is more than likely that arguments will occur. No relationship exists in a vacuum, and everyone experiences periods of intense stress. If, for example, in addition to the usual demands, you find yourself having to move just as you are planning for the arrival of your second child, and your mother-in-law is arranging a visit, you are likely to feel irritable and more than usually prone to argument. It helps to be as compassionate as possible with your love partner when going through a high-stress period.

If, in spite of your intention to stay calm, you find yourself irritable and angry when you or your lover are under stress, ask for a break. The purpose is not to avoid a necessary discussion but rather to take some time for each of you to relax and regain composure. You might say, "This argument is out of control and destructive. Let's take twenty minutes to cool down and unwind. Then we'll be calmer and more receptive to working it out." You also have the right to say, "Thanks for your input. I'd like to give it careful thought during a twenty-minute time-out and talk about it later."

This time-out is useful for exorcising rage privately and safely, whether you go for a brisk walk or sit down to meditate and relax. In any case, a time-out will help avoid adding fuel to feelings of self-righteousness or indignation. Your time-out is an opportunity to look at both sides of the issue and consider how you may have contributed to the problem, perhaps by repeating some negative pattern or unfairly venting your frustration on your love partner.

From the following list, select the areas in which you and your lover most frequently experience anxiety, conflict, and tension:

- Finances
- Child rearing
- Extended family, in-laws, ex-spouse
- Career vs. home
- Time management
- Sex and intimacy
- Personal habits—such as alcoholism or drug abuse

At a time when you are most relaxed, brainstorm creatively, looking for alternatives and choices that will reduce stress and eliminate the risk of a destructive argument. For example, you may choose to go out to dinner one less evening per week and apply the savings toward a housekeeper. Or take turns having special time with your children, freeing your spouse to explore leisurely interests—athletics, music, or reading.

As I have mentioned previously, most people assume they can accomplish more in a given period than is actually possible. You and your love partner would be wise in setting goals and deadlines to allow extra time for things to go wrong. You can also avoid unnecessary stress by setting personal and relationship priorities. In that way you can effectively plan which choices and commitments will take precedence in your lives.

ANXIETY-ANGER TRAP 8: ACCUSATIONS

Anxiety can lead to accusations. These expressions can range from subtle body language—raised eyebrows, a wagging finger, or shaking the head—to an out-of-control verbal attack: "What the hell's wrong with you?" Suppose your lover said to you in an accusing tone, "You don't love me." Your reaction would probably be defensive: "Sure I do. How can you say that? I tell you I love you all the time. What's the matter with you?" You don't really want to know what's behind those accusations or what your lover expects; you just want to talk your lover out of them because you feel so uncomfortable. You might even want to make him or her ashamed of the accusation. A lot of us are critical of our love partners for criticizing us! Unfortunately, this leads to a cycle of accusation—what you resist persists.

Accusations are a way of life in many relationships. Many people sincerely feel their lovers could improve by changing, so they berate continuously in the misguided belief that such criticism is helpful. An accusation such as "Damn it; do you have to be such a slob? What do you think I am, your mother?" is rarely met with "You're right, honey, from now on I'll put my clothes in the hamper." A common retort would be "Get off my back and stop being such a nag. You're always so uptight." When you and your lover get caught in escalating accusations, remind yourselves that mutual love is more important than determining who's at fault or who started the argument.

When you strive to be compassionate and understanding, you will ask questions with tenderness and curiosity. First determine whether your perception of the other person is correct: "I'd like to know more about what I've done that upsets you," or "You must have good reasons for feeling as you do. Please trust me with your anxiety, anger, or pain," or "What do you want that you're not getting now, that would give you the experience of being loved more deeply?"

When your lover is accusatory or angry with you, try to listen to the message of hurt and restrain the temptation to be defensive. This takes great strength, but once you understand your own anger and tendency to criticize, you can better accept your lover's anger and accusations. You can make constructive statements even if your love partner doesn't know how. Ask what you did to cause the hurt, what you can do to change, and what is necessary for the anger and accusations to subside.

ANXIETY-ANGER TRAP 9: "SHOULDS" AND "HAVE TO'S"

A love relationship built upon "shoulds" feels like a prison. Tight, raised shoulders are often the result. Burden your lover with "shoulds" and you create resistance and resentment rather than the satisfying freedom to love and serve. For a relationship to thrive, it is best for each partner to feel as if it's about 90 percent "want to's" and only about 10 percent "shoulds" and "have to's." Learning to say, "I would prefer it if—" instead of "You should—," or "It would be nice if—" as opposed to "You have to—" is a critical lesson in encouraging your lover to meet your needs. "Shoulds" and "have to's" trigger old resentments from childhood toward a critical parent.

Most people criticize their lovers for the things they fear and can't accept in themselves. For instance, if your partner accuses you of being lazy or sloppy, there is a good chance your actions have triggered a response of disapproval toward your lover's own laziness. Your lover is saying, "How can I possibly tolerate in you what I criticize myself for all the time?"

You may be inspired to improve your housecleaning habits, or you may be satisfied that you are already sufficiently hardworking, clean, and orderly. In either case, the more you recognize that your lover's demands reflect his or her own turmoil, the less likely you are to take those demands personally. In your love relationship, you mirror one another.

Instead of reacting defensively with "You're never satisfied with what I do around the house," empathize with your partner by saying, "A clean house is important to me also. Let's discuss what arrangement would be most satisfying for both of us." With this statement you are not out to vilify your partner but rather to look for a happy resolution that keeps the mirror clear and free of fear.

ANXIETY-ANGER TRAP 10: HITTING BELOW THE BELT

Partners in an intimate relationship know each other's most vulnerable points and levels of tolerance. Threats, warnings, and punishments—"If you do, I'll leave," "You'd better stop crying now"—produce fear and invite further retaliation and sabotage. Belt lines differ with each individual. Some lovers feel devastated by yelling and screaming; others cannot tolerate swearing or hostile silence.

Another low blow is invalidating your lover with inappropriate attacks:

"You're just hostile to men."
"You're a resentful mama's boy and woman-hater."
"You're crazy."
"You're a pathological liar."
"You must have done something to create that yourself."

Such psychobabble arouses further anger and defensiveness. These comments are neither helpful nor therapeutic, just thinly veiled name-calling. If you resort to low blows, you will have to live in a hostile climate. The tendency to strike below the belt is another habit usually learned from watching parental arguments.

Now that you've identified the anxiety-anger traps that trouble your relationship, focus on making specific changes. A simple program of reminders can be very helpful. For example, one client placed copies of the following list on the nightstand, the car dashboard, and a kitchen bulletin board to help correct faulty tactics for dealing with conflict. It read:

ANXIETY-ANGER TRAPS TO WORK ON

- Don't anxiously mind read; never assume you know what your partner is thinking or feeling. Ask instead of tell.
- Avoid "you are" messages and use "I feel" messages instead. For example, say, "I feel ignored and unappreciated when you don't call and come home late." Don't say, "You are a hostile and selfish s.o.b. for always being late."
- Don't blame, complain, accuse, label, or attack. Listen, praise, compliment, and forgive.

Make up your own list to carry in your pocket, place by your bed, or put on your refrigerator door to assist you in learning new, positive habits for handling anger and communicating your needs. These reminders will help you reduce anxiety in your intimate relationships and improve communication skills on a daily basis.

Carl Jung taught that "everything that irritates us about others can lead us to an understanding of ourselves." The people you react to most strongly, whether with love, fear, or hate, are projections of your inner state. Stretch your awareness by observing the mirror of relationship. The single most important strategy to head off defensive communication is to consciously choose to hold on to a positive, loving image of your partner and keep reintroducing praise and admiration into your relationship.

28

Healing the Anxiety of Loss and Change

Heavy thoughts bring on physical maladies.
—MARTIN LUTHER

In an era of quick fixes and instant gratification, no one wants to talk about the anxiety that results from heartbreak. With the American worship of winning, many people believe that to admit loss, or the fear of losing, is a sign of weakness, immaturity, and failure. The wholesale denial of loss contributes to the epidemic of anxiety and depression.

The elderly are twice as likely as the general population to suffer from depression. One reason is the greater frequency of loss in this age group. The death of a spouse, friend, or family member, poor health, retirement, financial problems, relocation to a retirement community or nursing home, and confronting their own mortality are just some of the losses dealt with by people in the final chapters of their lives. Studies show that as we age, serotonin declines and cortisol levels rise. The result is often chronically high levels of stress among the elderly, and for those who are especially vulnerable, anxiety and depression. There is no segment of the population for whom benzodiazepine tranquilizers are more overprescribed than for the elderly. Too often these pills just compound their problems.

The relationship between the onset of anxiety and the occurrence of loss is well researched. Anxiety, stress, and often illness tend to occur around significant life events, transitions, and crises in people's lives. Create a "lifeline"—a chart on which you note the major losses, changes, and turning points in your life. Is there an association between the onset of periods of anxiety and your major life changes?

In studying the relationship between life changes and bouts of anxiety and illness, psychiatrists Thomas H. Holmes and Richard H. Rahe attempted to depict this correlation more exactly by measuring the severity of change in the period before the illness. Of course, no two people respond identically to the same change or loss. Following a divorce, death of a close friend, or loss of a job, one person may have only mild feelings of anxiety and depression, while someone else may develop an anxiety disorder or major depression.

Holmes and Rahe did research among people of different countries, social classes, and ages and came up with forty-three common life changes, with their relative adaptive demands given a score on a scale from 1 to 100. Their Social Readjustment Rating Scale, published originally in 1967 in the *Journal of Psychosomatic Research*, was as follows:

LIFE EVENT	MEAN VALUE
· Death of spouse	100
· Divorce	73
· Marital separation	65
· Detention in jail or other institution	63
· Death of a close family member	63
· Major personal injury or illness	53

LIFE EVENT	MEAN VALUE
· Marriage	50
· Being fired at work	47
· Marital reconciliation	45
· Retirement from work	45
· Major change in the health or behavior of a family member	44
· Pregnancy	40
· Sexual difficulties	39
· Gaining a new family member through birth, adoption, oldster moving in, etc.	39
· Major business readjustment, such as a merger, reorganization, bankruptcy, etc.	39
· Major change in financial state	38
· Death of a close friend	37
· Changing to a different line of work	36
· Major change in the number of arguments with spouse	35
· Taking on a mortgage, such as purchasing a home, business, etc.	31
· Foreclosure on a mortgage or loan	30
· Major change in responsibilities at work, such as promotion, demotion, lateral transfer	29
· Son or daughter leaving home for marriage, attending college, etc.	29
· In-law troubles	29
· Outstanding personal achievement	28
· Wife beginning or ceasing work outside the home	26
· Beginning or ceasing formal schooling	26
· Major change in living conditions	25
· Revision of personal habits	24
· Troubles with the boss	23
· Major change in working hours or conditions	20
· Change in residence	20
· Changing to a new school	20
· Major change in usual type and/or amount of recreation	19

LIFE EVENT	MEAN VALUE
· Major change in spiritual beliefs or religious affiliation	19
· Major change in social activities	18
· Taking on a mortgage or loan less than $10,000	17
· Major change in sleeping habits	16
· Major change in number of family get-togethers	15
· Major change in eating habits	13
· Vacation	13
· Christmas	12
· Minor violations of the law, such as a traffic ticket, jaywalking, disturbing the peace, etc.	11

Apply the Holmes-Rahe scale to yourself. Check off each of the life events on the chart that happened to you during the year immediately preceding either your current or last significant bout with anxiety. If an event occurred twice in that year, it should be checked twice. The corresponding number values for the changes in that year should then be added up, providing your total score for the life changes and losses you experienced during that time period.

Since developing their original scale, Holmes and his colleagues have suggested that people assign their own readjusted values to their life changes. So go back over the scale, and estimate for yourself, compared to their scale of 1 to 100, how much each life change demanded or took out of you. For example, if you had a particularly horrific, contentious divorce, you might give yourself a score of 80 or 85 instead of the suggested 73 for the average divorce. Then recalculate your total score according to your own estimates. This will give you a more personally accurate reflection of the demands and losses you have faced.

Research on anxiety and stress has shown that the severity of the disorder is often correlated with a higher score on this scale. A higher incidence of physical illnesses, from diabetes to tuberculosis, has been associated with higher Social

Readjustment scores. Even the incidence of accidents has been correlated with higher scores. Notice on the Holmes-Rahe scale that ten of the fifteen most challenging life events are associated with marriage and family (e.g., death of a spouse or family member, divorce, marriage, marital separation). This shows the importance of marital and family relationships to both emotional and physical health. It may be true that a person can literally die of a broken heart!

Knowledge of the scale can help you heal anxiety and prevent future recurrences. Become familiar with the life events and the amount of relative adjustment they require. Using this as a guide enables you to predict potential sources of difficulty. For example, let's assume you're currently suffering from anxiety and considering taking on a hefty mortgage or relocating to another city to begin a new career. Based upon your understanding of the stress that may be involved, you might defer these changes until after you have healed. Even if you decide to go for it, you will be better able to anticipate and prepare for the inner demands of these changes. You could, for instance, take a meditation course as part of a strategy to leave extra time for self-care.

THE STAGES OF HEALING

The top three items on the Holmes-Rahe scale are death of a spouse, divorce, and marital separation. Natural self-healing of your emotions means recognizing that a broken heart requires at least as much care and compassion as a broken leg. What follows are knowledge and strategies for dealing with a major loss.[1]

There are two constants in life: love and loss. Following a loss, anxiety and depression are perfectly natural. What few people realize is that a major loss inflicts an emotional wound that requires just as much care and attention to heal properly as a serious physical injury. After even a minor cut, you wash it and put on a Band-Aid. A broken back may require weeks in the hospital and months before full function is restored. A major emotional loss requires just as much care and time to heal properly. If you don't know how to treat the emotional wounds of loss, the sad result can be slow healing and unnecessary emotional damage.

Just as the body goes through stages in healing a physical wound, the mind passes through three recognizable stages in its recovery from loss. First come shock and denial. Unable to cope with a sudden emotional blow, the mind temporarily blocks it out. We say things to ourselves such as "I can't believe it!" "He couldn't have done such a thing!" "This isn't happening!" or we just feel numb. After a major loss there may be complete emotional paralysis lasting from a few moments to a few months.

When the shock begins to wear off, the second stage gradually unfolds. This is the period of fear, anger, and depression. Whenever you're hurt by someone you love or trust, anger is an automatic and completely natural response, as is depression. A loss is a major threat to your well-being. Anxiety and crying are natural. The key to moving on from this stage is fully experiencing the pain and fear and allowing expression of the anger without any guilt. This is where the healing often gets stuck.

Once the pain is fully felt and the anger vented, the loss becomes a fact that can be accepted and understood. With enough time, it becomes less devastating. It is a painful event, but you survived. Energy and strength gradually return, often in greater measure than before.

EMOTIONAL FIRST AID

Following a major loss, the first response is anxiety and help-lessness. Out of tragic disappointment and bottomless frustration, it's very easy to fall into a cycle of self-punishment. Some people punish themselves by repeatedly going over the event in their minds, constantly telling themselves, "If only I had done something different." But nothing can be changed. Loss leaves you feeling helpless.

TEN DO'S AND DON'TS FOR A BROKEN HEART

DO'S	DON'TS
Stay calm; treat yourself gently.	Don't panic.
Recognize your injury.	Don't deny the hurt.
Be with the pain.	Don't blame yourself.
Take time to heal.	Don't dwell on the negative.
Rest, nurture yourself.	Don't abuse alcohol or drugs.
Accept comfort from friends and family.	Don't stay isolated.
Stick to a routine.	Don't create more chaos.
Take care in making important decisions.	Don't make impulsive judgments; be wary of love on the rebound.
Accept understanding and support.	Don't be afraid to ask for help.
Anticipate a positive outcome.	Don't lose faith.

You can't change the past, but the next best thing is to learn what you *can* change and make your pain serve your growth. The strategies for coping with loss are divided into three groups, corresponding to the three stages of healing.

1. SHOCK AND DENIAL

You can't believe it happened. You feel numb, disoriented, help-less. All these feelings are OK too. The struggle to believe and disbelieve your loss simultaneously is natural. Give it time. The loss is real. Let yourself accept the reality that the worst has happened. Don't try to deny it. Even small losses and dis-appointments, like losing a quarter in a pay phone, hurt a little. Big losses hurt a lot. The fact that you can be disappointed and hurting is proof that you're human. It's natural to be fright-ened of pain at first. Sometimes it can get so bad that it threat-ens to swallow you up. Don't panic or start fighting it. Lean gently into your pain. You won't find it bottomless.

Loss is a blow to your self-esteem. Your worry, self-con-demnation, and self-deprecation are symptoms of your loss, nothing more. They have only temporary reality. Don't give them prime-time status by paying them much attention. Better to tell yourself that you're strong enough to go on and trans-form your loss into something better. Beware of the "if only's." Every time you punish yourself with what you might have done, you fall for the trap of trying to make believe that the past can be changed. It can't. "If only's" don't count, so don't use them.

Remember that a loss is just as much a wound as a cut or a broken bone. It hurts, and you have to give it time to heal. More than anything else, you need plenty of time. You can be confident that you will heal. The same powerful healing forces that can mend a broken bone also mend the emotional trauma of a loss. Take heart, nature is on your side.

The greater the loss, the more time you'll take to heal. In this era of instant gratification, many people are unwilling to give themselves the time they need. Don't make this costly mis-take. Time may be a luxury, but you deserve it. Be careful not to rush your healing, or the result will be chronic strain. Real healing results in a new feeling of ease and appreciation for life. The healing process is not smooth. You're going to have ups and downs. One day you may feel the pain is almost gone; the next day you seem to hurt as much as ever. Don't worry about ups and downs. They're a sign that healing is under way.

2. FEAR, ANGER, AND DEPRESSION

Cry. Don't believe that old sexist stuff about men not crying. If you hurt and the tears are coming, let them come. Tears are cleansing and serve the healing process by letting you fully feel your pain. Crying is an important and natural form of release. It has its own beauty. You are more fragile now, there is no shame in that, so take it easy. Don't hurry. Don't try to force yourself to do things like going to parties or to the movies when you don't want to. Ask a friend to come over for a quiet evening of music and talk. Avoid stressful situations that might force you to overreact. Now is not the time to take on new responsibilities. Tread slowly for a while. You deserve the special care.

Thinking of him or her? If you have lost a love through divorce or separation, it's natural to dream about rekindling the relationship. But a forceful hand is best. Imagining that you can renew a relationship once it's over is another form of "if only." It's self-punishment, like pouring salt on an open wound. The only result is more pain. Don't indulge in self-punishment. Nothing is more painful than accepting the fact that a love relationship is over. Accept it now, face the realities, let yourself hurt. That's the way to healing, growth, and a greater capacity for love in the future.

Release your anger. Everyone who suffers a loss or disappointment gets angry. Some may have trouble showing it, others difficulty in controlling it. But the anger is inevitable. To recover from your loss, you have to get the anger out. The biggest obstacle to healing is bottled-up anger.

Pamper yourself. Were you to suffer from a broken leg, you'd find friends and relatives bringing you fruit and candy to cheer you up. Though you've suffered an emotional wound that's just as serious, you're expected to show up for work every day as if nothing had happened. You live in a world that doesn't acknowledge that emotional wounds hurt badly. The only way to fight back is to pamper yourself. Take a hot herbal bath, get a massage, buy yourself something you would really enjoy, get a manicure or pedicure.

Let go of your pain. Paradoxically, pain can become a friend. You may be tempted to hold on to it longer than necessary. The unconscious thinking goes something like "I've lost something really important to me, but at least I have my pain." The pain itself becomes a source of stability, albeit unhappy. At some point your pain will gradually slip away. Let it go. Only then can you go on to the next step, where surviving your loss begins to pay off. You discover the new you, more powerful, more loving, and wiser than before.

Heal at your own pace. Friends or relatives may tell you, "It's about time you got over it" or "That's enough crying. Now you'd better get on with your life." This advice is well intentioned, but remember that you have the right to experience your pain fully and to live through each stage of the healing process fully. Telling yourself, "It doesn't matter" or "I'm all right now" when you don't feel that way is a phony attempt to move on prematurely to the stage of acceptance and understanding. If you've suffered a major loss, it may take a year or more before you have really reached the stage of acceptance. Not that your life has stopped in the interim, but you have the right to take it a little easier during that time, to pamper yourself and mourn at your own pace.

3. ACCEPTANCE AND GROWTH

Now is the time to begin transforming your loss into personal growth. As the pain lessens, your thinking becomes sharper, your judgment grows clearer, your concentration improves, and you begin to be less self-preoccupied. Your feelings are more alive. You are stronger. There's no reason to settle for just putting the past behind you. You can learn from it and discover new inner strengths.

Forgive. Whether your lover left you, your friends betrayed you, your boss fired you, or fate dealt you a bad break, you gain strength by forgiving as soon as you can. Remember, you don't forgive for the other person's benefit but for your own. Also, forgiving does not mean forgetting. To forgive originally meant "to return good treatment for ill usage." You have been ill used. When you can return good feeling toward the person who injured you, you are finally free. Forgive yourself. OK, you made a mistake. Maybe things would be different now if you had done something else, but there is no point in punishing yourself any further. Forgiving yourself is acceptance and a step toward freedom and wisdom.

Try to begin seeing the positive in your loss. Yes, there is something positive. You've learned something about the world and yourself. Perhaps you were naive, or didn't understand how complicated love relationships can become, or how people change, or how ruthless the business world can be. The point is: your loss is an extraordinary opportunity for rapid growth. Take advantage of it by examining why you lost and what you need to do to avoid making the same mistake in the future.

Accept that you're a better person for having loved and lost than if you had never loved at all. You became involved; you took a risk and chose to love. You aren't a coward. All of that speaks well of you. Now you are stronger for having lived through your disappointment and learned from it.

Give of yourself. The only way to begin using your new strength is to start flexing your muscles. You're not so fragile anymore; you can take risks, share your feelings, trust yourself to love again. Start by sharing yourself in small ways. Offer to help a friend with a project; volunteer to help at a hospital or nursing home; drive an elderly person to the grocery store. When someone asks you about yourself, you don't have to protect yourself. There's no need for a mask. You know what the world is about, and you can handle it. The greatest joys are in sharing your real feelings. Let yourself get involved. Take hold of your new freedom.

You know much more now about yourself and about others. No longer must you react to the world; you can create the world you want to live in. No longer are you so dependent on others; you can choose when, where, how, and with whom you want to spend time. You can choose one of your dreams and take the careful steps to make it come true. No longer do you need to hold yourself back out of fear of failure or loss; you've been healed. Make new friends. At long last you're ready to begin pursuing your life at full swing. Have the neighbors over for a drink. Join a health club or social group where you will meet new people. Don't be afraid to be friendly.

THE LOSS OF SAFETY

It is through being wounded that power grows and can, in the end, become tremendous.
—FRIEDRICH NIETZSCHE

A traumatic assault can strike suddenly, but its emotional pain can last for years. No matter how healthy you are, grief from a traumatic attack can cause profound distress that's as painful as any experience life can bring. Difficult as it is, however, grieving can't be avoided or hurried. Natural healing takes time and patience.

After an attack, such as rape, battery, or assault, grief usually runs a long and tortuous route—anxiety, fears, sleep disorders, rage, loss of appetite, crying, preoccupation with objects and locations associated with the attack, and crushed hopes and dreams.

Survivors often feel unsafe in their bodies. Their emotions and thinking feel out of control. They also feel unsafe in relation to other people. These post-traumatic stresses can be treated in a variety of ways, such as with herbal or synthetic medicines to reduce fear and anxiety, cognitive-behavioral therapy, meditation, and vigorous exercise to help manage stress.

Cognitive-behavioral strategies consist of the recognition and naming of symptoms, daily logs to chart symptoms and adaptive responses, the identification and implementation of manageable "homework" assignments, and specific comprehensive safety plans—at home, when traveling, and at work.

The traumatized person needs a guaranteed safe refuge, either at home or in a secured shelter. The damage to safety in relationships must be addressed with progressive interpersonal strategies, such as the gradual development of a trusting relationship in psychotherapy or counseling, and social strategies that mobilize the survivor's natural support system of family and friends. The task of reestablishing safety is especially complex when the survivor is still involved in a relationship that has been abusive in the past. The potential for violence should always be considered, even if the survivor insists he or she is no longer afraid.

Establishing a safe environment requires more than just the mobilization of caring people. It requires the assessment of continued threat and exactly what precautions are sensible or necessary. For example, housing and counseling at a shelter for battered women may be necessary while the threat of continued danger is assessed.

One may not reach the dawn save by the path of the night.

—KAHLIL GIBRAN

As recovery from a traumatic attack proceeds, the survivor needs to find ways to tell the story of the trauma, completely, in depth, and with detail. This grief work helps the traumatic memory so that it can be integrated into the survivor's life story.

Survivors of traumatic attack should be encouraged to turn to others for support, but considerable care must be taken to ensure that they choose people they can truly trust. Family members, friends, lovers, and close friends may be of immense help, or they may interfere with recovery or be dangerous themselves. A careful evaluation must be made of each important relationship in a traumatized person's life, assessing each as a source of potential protection, emotional support, practical help, and also as a possible source of danger.

Identify whatever feels best to you for finding solace during times of grief. For some, spending time outdoors in a natural setting is uplifting. For others, hurts are resolved best by browsing through photo albums or old letters. Express your feelings of grief. This may mean talking with loved ones, close friends, and perhaps your family physician or counselor. You might also find it beneficial to talk with those who have experienced similar losses, by joining an organized support group for victims of violent crimes.

A technique called eye movement desensitization and reprocessing (EMDR) has proven effective for post-traumatic stress disorder in seventeen controlled studies. The EMDR patient is asked to recall the traumatic event while performing rapid eye movements back and forth. This process is thought to help the brain "metabolize" the painful memories.

HEALING THE PAIN
OF CHILDHOOD

Happiness is having a large, loving, caring, close-knit family in another city.

—GEORGE BURNS

Adult anxieties can have their roots in the losses—rejection, betrayal, humiliation, neglect, and terror—of childhood. The loving, innocent heart of a child has little protection other than to suppress fear, shame, and pain in the deep recesses of the psyche. Sigmund Freud described the *repetition compulsion:* whatever was experienced as traumatic, deficient, or incomplete in your childhood, there is a tendency to recreate. When a child feels deeply intimidated, hurt, or rejected, this may begin a lifetime struggle with anxiety.

Whatever your age, to become a fulfilled person and be at peace, you must resolve the issues that derived from your relationships with your parents.[2] Below are the warning signs that unhealed emotional wounds from childhood may be contributing to your adult anxieties:

- You create an arm's-length-only intimacy for fear of being trapped in a committed love relationship or marriage.
- You find yourself experiencing the same money or health fears a parent had.
- You find yourself reenacting upsetting events or upheavals from childhood.
- You frequently feel emotionally abused, like a victim or martyr.
- You suffer from fears of rejection, disapproval, or abandonment.
- You feel left out, overlooked, unappreciated, or taken for granted at home or at work.

Although there may be an innate tendency to repeat your childhood dramas, you can also work through them. What you need is an understanding of how your upbringing affected you, what negative attitudes you may have internalized, and how to change these outdated emotional habits. The Hoffman Quadrinity Process (HQP)[3] is a one-week intensive residential program that guides participants through deep and rapid healing of the roots of anxiety in all four aspects of self—physical, emotional, intellectual, and spiritual. The HQP was a profound breakthrough in my own healing journey and subsequently for hundreds of my patients.

RESILIENCY—
RISING ABOVE ADVERSITY

When one door closes, another opens. But we often look so long and so regretfully upon the closed door that we do not see the one which has opened for us.
                                                    —HELEN KELLER

Resiliency is the ability to rise above serious loss and adversity—the inner strength to master change successfully. A potentially stressful event, such as a financial setback, will have a different impact on different individuals depending on their resiliency. One person may find the stress of a minor fender-bender to be a nightmare, while someone else seriously injured in an auto accident remains emotionally stable, forgiving, and optimistic. The stress incurred depends not only on the life event but on the resiliency of the individual.

Aspects of resiliency include a sense of being in control, the ability to make your own decisions, and having good coping skills. A high rate of hypertension and heart disease has been linked to job strain, where employees feel highly pressured but have little control over how they meet job demands. The ability to cope with job strain, such as that from corporate down-sizing, business recessions, and new technologies, is affected by the strength of your business and social networks. Research has demonstrated that support from family, friends, coworkers, and even pets can act as a buffer in coping with strains at work. Intimate relationships can help shore up self-esteem that is temporarily lost and provide comfort during turbulent times in the workplace.

LOVING FRIENDS

How we approach other people each day can determine whether we experience isolation, chronic stress, suffering, and illness, or intimacy, relaxation, joy, and health.
                                          —DEAN ORNISH, M.D.

There is a vital link between the strength of your social support system and your resilience to loss of any kind. Simply having a close friend to talk to on a regular basis may be as important as psychotherapy. Deep, caring relationships really do matter; isolation increases human anxiety. *Social support* is the name scientists give to the combination of ongoing involvement with others, caring relationships, and an orientation toward actively seeking friendships. Social support doesn't depend on the number of people you know but rather on the quality of your relationships.

Take a sheet of paper and write down the names of those people with whom you have the strongest, closest bond. Include those who have been sources of warmth and approval during earlier periods of your life as well as those who actively support you now. As you list the names, you may find yourself wishing you were in closer touch with some of them.

If so, list these people on a second sheet of paper. Entries may include old friends you haven't seen in a long time or new friends you'd like to get to know better.

Now make a list of what you would like to discuss with each friend. There may be some people with or for whom you would like to do something special—meet for lunch, or send a letter or gift to let them know they're really important to you. Is there anyone you'd like to call right now?

HELPING OTHERS HELPS YOURSELF

We make a living by what we get, but we make a life by what we give.

—SIR WINSTON CHURCHILL

Studies clearly suggest that a weekly habit of helping others may be as important to your health and longevity as regular exercise and good nutrition. In fact, it may be a key to ending the deadly cycle of fear, loneliness, and depression rampant in our society. Medical research indicates that self-centered individuals have a greater risk of anxiety, depression, and even coronary artery disease. Self-involvement breeds fear, loneliness, and despair. Altruism, charity, generosity, service, and kindness contribute not only to a meaningful life but to a more satisfying, healthier, and perhaps longer one as well. Doing good for others feels good and is good for your own well-being. Love can bolster your resistance to disease and speed the healing of anxiety.

Focusing on others gets you out of the gridlock of career anxieties, financial worries, and family stresses. Helping others tends to improve mood, deepen optimism, and nurture a genuine sense of gratitude. Helping someone less capable can enhance your appreciation of your own skills, knowledge, and strengths. Contrary to popular opinion, helping others doesn't require a huge time commitment. All you need is a personal plan that can range from doing scheduled work with a volunteer organization to spontaneous acts of generosity and kindness throughout the week. Joining an anxiety self-help support group is a wonderful way to help yourself and also contribute to helping others (see Appendix E).

Much research has shown that helping, caring relationships can diminish anxiety and improve health. A study of 2,700 residents in Tecumseh, Michigan, demonstrated that men who did volunteer work were two-and-a-half times less likely to die from all causes of disease than their peers who were not engaged in service. A lack of social support and community service is a health risk factor as significant as smoking, elevated cholesterol, and sedentary living.

Spiritual Crisis and Renewing Your Soul

We are not human beings having a spiritual experience. We are spiritual beings having a human experience.
—PIERRE TEILHARD DE CHARDIN

Anxiety may signal a crisis not only of body and mind but also of spirit. Your anxiety may be energy in search of greater adventure and purpose. What do you want from life? What do you value? What do you find most satisfying and meaningful? What is your purpose? Though your world may seem in turmoil, a deeper sense of understanding and inspiration is trying to emerge. A crisis of meaning is not just a breakdown but an opportunity for your spirit to break through. It may seem paradoxical, but a spiritual crisis can serve to improve your life dramatically.

For a lot of people today, a crisis of meaning and purpose seems to be precipitated by a discrepancy between the work they do and their personal values. For more and more people, the basic issue is no longer mere survival but living with integrity. The challenge is no longer living up to other people's expectations but discovering a deeper purpose and satisfaction. For such people the driving motivation is no longer "How do I make the most money or rise above my peers?" but "What will give meaning to my life?"

SEEKING AUTHENTICITY AND INTEGRITY

The great malady of the twentieth century ... is loss of soul. When the soul is neglected, it doesn't just go away; it appears in obsessions, addictions, violence, and loss of meaning. If the soul's capacity for creativity is not honored it will wreak havoc.

—THOMAS MOORE

One way to discover how you may be sacrificing your integrity is to examine the difference between how you present yourself to others and your true feelings. People who repeatedly suppress their true self in favor of a false image, act, or facade end up feeling phony, dishonest, controlled, superficial, plastic, or "always on display." They are constantly rehearsing what they are about to say and criticizing the phoniness of what they just said. They also become increasingly resentful of their compliance and of those whom they try to impress.

If you have been compromising your values, you may find yourself filled with rationalizations like "If I didn't do it, someone else would," "It's the only way to get ahead," or "You can't fight the system." Eventually you may find yourself cut off from your emotions, defensive with friends and loved ones, and only half-hearted about your success. Tired of straining and pretending, you desire to be more authentic but are afraid to let down the facade. The discrepancy between your Natural Self (see chapter 21) and the social role you play results in anxiety.

In contrast, when you are inspired to live by your deepest values, you are more likely to feel free, spontaneous, and alive. Instead of feeling that everything is a burden or that everyone is judging you, your emotions lighten up and your work becomes more meaningful. When you strive to do your best at something you value, you stop worrying about how you compare with others. You are more likely to appreciate your own goodness and the goodness of others and to enjoy being acknowledged not just for what you do but for who you are. There is no greater opportunity than to commit to your highest vision and live your life courageously.

If you feel you don't understand the spiritual dimension of your personality and aren't prepared to cope with your spiritual needs, a spiritual crisis can be terrifying. But like all crises that accompany transitions, a spiritual crisis is also an opportunity for personal growth.

DRAWING OUT YOUR SHADOW

A spiritual crisis can be terrifying because it can suddenly generate an abyss of anxiety. Our *shadow* is where we put our disowned thoughts, feelings, and behaviors. At midlife, it is where our inner demons and monsters lie in wait. Making peace with your dark side, what Mother Teresa called her inner Hitler, is an imperative on the spiritual path. The dread of the "dark night of the soul" can be rough. Sooner or later each of us gets driven, literally or figuratively, to our knees. The only question is whether it is through *humility*, surrendering to a higher power, or *humiliation*, clinging to egotistical control.

In spiritual psychology, the shadow refers to the dark side of the human personality, the dreaded rage and jealousy that lie buried within the unconscious. If your shadow side remains unexplored and untamed, it is all too easy to project your disowned lying, selfish, and vindictive tendencies onto others. To make peace with yourself, you must face and own your own shadow. You must come to grips with the inner enemy you have been so ashamed of and so reviled. When you see someone else as inferior, immoral, disgusting, or psychopathic, turn the mirror around onto yourself to see what you can learn about your shadow.

A helpful exercise is *drawing out your shadow*. Draw images, with paint or crayons on canvas or on paper, that symbolize the disowned and uncomfortable parts of yourself, the parts you generally choose to hide. Focus on pure emotional expression rather than the normal concerns of art, with no critical editing of your visions. The simple act of drawing is healing because it takes shadow feelings that have felt out of control and gives them a conscious image. If painful or frightening images come up, keep drawing. Later you may also try drawing a healing light to surround these images.

Drawing pictures can help you learn more about the inner projections of your shadow. First close your eyes to fully experience the negative feelings you harbor. When the negativity has reached a peak of intensity, start to draw your rage, hatred, or disgust on paper while your eyes are still closed. When it feels right, open your eyes and continue to draw, using different colors and images to vent any cruel, murderous, or abhorrent feelings. Feelings and old memories may come up that you have been repressing for a lifetime.

Drawing is a creative way to exorcise your demons. If you don't feel safe with this process, you might consider doing appropriate shadow work with a trained mental health professional. Far from being merely a black bag of darkness, the shadow holds the key to the lost depths of your soul.[1]

FACING YOUR MORTALITY

Caution: If you currently suffer from suicidal thoughts, severe anxiety, or panic attacks, these exercises may not be appropriate for you unless done under the supervision or guidance of a mental health professional.

Underlying your anxiety may be a fear of death. Facing and accepting your own mortality may be uncomfortable at first, but it can be an enormously liberating experience. No matter how healthy you become, death is inevitable. Acknowledging the inevitability of death can make us whole. As Montaigne wrote, "Facing death teaches us to live." By confronting and mourning your own mortality, you can begin to see through the eyes of your soul.

Please handle the following questions and exercises with caution. Take some uninterrupted time to imagine your own death. What are your worst fears? What would you want to say to each of your loved ones, friends and family, before you die? Use mental imagery to visualize your funeral service. What do family and friends say about the role you played, or failed to play, in their lives? How do you feel about what they say? What would you want to change about how you related to them? Take some time to write your own obituary. Envision the specific kinds of qualities, actions, and contributions to the world for which you want to be remembered. Facing your own mortality is not easy, but it is a surefire way to focus more attention on your spiritual self and heartfelt values.

There is an old story that Plato, on his deathbed, was asked by a friend if he would summarize his life's great works, the dialogues, in one statement. Plato, coming out of a reverie, looked at his friend and said, "Practice dying." Your journey does not begin or end in the material world. A spiritual crisis can awaken you to the immortality of your soul. Spirit is nature's healing energy and wholeness, the eternal flow of creative intelligence in every cell of your body. As the great Chinese poet Chang-Tzu wrote, "That which fills the universe I regard as my body, and that which directs the universe I see as my own nature."

The fear of death—its inevitability and finality, its grotesque mysteriousness—is perhaps the source of more misery for more people than anything else. There is ample evidence that hopelessness, loss of meaning, and an impending sense of doom are toxic to the body in many ways. These emotions often accompany our attitudes toward death. Today we know they exert a depressant effect on the body's immune function and can set in motion irreversible, sometimes fatal processes in the heart and circulatory system as well. Thus it is no exaggeration to say that our attitude toward death literally can be a matter of life and death.

—LARRY DOSSEY, M.D.

NURTURING YOUR SOUL

A spiritual life of some kind is essential for emotional well-being. Your philosophy of life or faith in a higher power—your spirituality—considerably influences your mental health. Albert Einstein said that we often suffer from a kind of optical delusion in acting as if we're not connected to life in all of its forms. This separateness is the most painful delusion on earth and underlies much anxiety. To nurture your soul, consider the following.

- *Spend time alone:* Spiritual growth is almost impossible if you never give yourself a chance to explore your own thoughts and feelings in private. If you have avoided time alone, your initial efforts to do so may result in some anxiety. Put that anxiety into a task that expresses your innermost feelings. You could write poetry, paint, take photographs, or go for a walk in the woods.

Once you make a habit of spending time alone, you will treasure solitude because you will have discovered how nourishing it is for your soul. You will also realize that fulfillment lies within yourself. You can never find fulfillment in someone else, but you can share it once you have found it within.

- *Attend to your spiritual growth:* Whether you prefer the Bible or Walt Whitman, you can learn much by studying what others have written about spiritual development. At the very least you will gain the reassurance that spiritual angst is a universal part of human experience.

  Strengthen your religious ties. Bible study classes and meditation retreats can provide an atmosphere and a community for exploration of eternal questions. You might also learn to pray, if you do not already pray regularly. Prayer can sometimes work miracles, so it can certainly heal anxiety. Clearly prayer can be a great comfort and a source of strength during times of stress.

- *Ponder the big unanswered questions of life:* For example, take time to drive out into the country on a clear night and look at the sky. Ask yourself where it all came from, how it keeps going, whether there is a divine plan. Or take a walk by the ocean and let yourself muse about the purpose of life. Don't lapse into cynicism, which is too easy. Existential questions can provoke anxiety, and cynicism is a common defense. Be open to the possibility that these questions may indeed have real answers that you can discover. Your goal should not be to find some absolute answer that you can follow as a new religion but simply to develop a personal philosophy of life that will nurture and sustain you. Seek and you shall find.

- *Seek pastoral counseling:* If you seek professional guidance in navigating your spiritual crisis, you need to find a counselor with some special skills. Above all, your counselor must be sensitive to the issues and dynamics of spiritual growth as well as those of ordinary emotional illness. The counselor you seek need not be a psychiatrist or psychologist. Your priest, rabbi, or minister may be very helpful, especially if he or she has been trained in pastoral counseling.

A well-trained pastoral counselor will not encourage you to repress your inner turmoil by adopting a set of prefabricated beliefs but instead will help you bring your feelings to the surface and discover your deepest needs. In addition, pastoral counselors are already intimately familiar with issues related to spiritual growth. They can assist you in Bible study and learning how to pray. These traditional activities may lead you to a renewed faith in God. Ultimately, this renewed religious faith will lead to a renewed faith in yourself.

To locate a pastoral counselor, contact your local church, synagogue, or hospital. If you feel the need for help during a spiritual crisis, don't hesitate to seek it. Spiritual upheaval is a natural part of living, and you shouldn't feel ashamed because you have deep doubts about the purpose and direction of your life.

PERSONAL AND
SOCIAL TRANSFORMATION

Love is the pursuit of the whole.

—Plato

Current research indicates that a spiritual crisis during midlife may be a necessary step toward discovery of inner creative resources that can bring renewal to the second half of your life. Through a successful resolution of a spiritual crisis, you can give up hidden childhood legacies of fear and anxiety that block the full blossoming of your talents. In many cases this process may involve a major life adjustment, such as resignation from an unsatisfying job or starting a new career. Initially difficult and sometimes painful, these steps can lead to a future of greater personal fulfillment.

The spiritual journey upon which your anxiety may have launched you can lead to more personal satisfaction and peace of mind but also something more. Healing anxiety changes your perception of yourself and your relationship to the world. As you become more aware of your personal power, you'll develop more empathy for every human being. This transformation will build on itself. The more you heal, the more you appreciate the inner dimension of your being, committing you to making a difference in the world.

Disapproving of those who try to solve social problems without attending to their inner lives, Socrates admonished, "Let him who would move the world first move himself." What he might have added is that once you do change yourself, changing the world becomes a biological and psychological imperative. This is significant in view of the criticism of the integrative health, human potential, and personal growth movements as promoting self-absorption at the expense of social commitment. While the pursuit of personal growth may require self-knowledge, the flowering of the personality comes from contributing to others.

In an attempt to control and dominate our way to health, we have disregarded our spiritual nature. Our collective psychology has suffered from epidemic levels of anxiety, stress, and depression because we have lost touch with the healing power of Mother Nature, including her marvelous herbal medicines. These potent remedies bring natural love and creative intelligence directly to heal our nervous system. Herbal medicines and natural self-healing can help us transcend our separation anxiety and become whole again. Attunement to natural herbal medicines allows us to rediscover the lost paradise of earth, and to humbly honor and respect our evolutionary place in the web of life.

APPENDIX A:
BIBLIOTHERAPY

A good book can be worth more than a dozen sessions. Many excellent self-help books can be used to facilitate progress in therapy.

—ARNOLD A. LAZARUS, PH.D.

Bloomfield, H. H., and Cooper, R. K. *The Power of 5*. Emmaus, Pa.: Rodale Press, 1995.

———. *Think Safe, Be Safe*. New York: Crown, 1997.

Bloomfield, H. H. and Felder, L. *Making Peace with Your Parents*. New York: Ballantine, 1984.

———. *Making Peace with Yourself*. New York: Ballantine, 1986.

Bloomfield, H. H., and Kory, R. B. *Inner Joy*. New York: Berkley, 1980.

Bloomfield, H. H., and McWilliams, P. *How to Heal Depression*. Los Angeles: Prelude Press, 1994.

Bloomfield, H. H., Nordfors, M., and McWilliams, P. *Hypericum and Depression*. Los Angeles: Prelude Press, 1996.

Bloomfield, H. H., Vettese, S., and Kory, R. B. *Lifemates*. New York: New American Library, 1989.

Borysenko, J. *Minding the Body, Mending the Mind*. Boston: Addison-Wesley, 1987.

Colgrove, M., Bloomfield, H. H., and McWilliams, P. *How to Survive the Loss of a Love*. Los Angeles: Prelude Press, 1992.

Concept: Synergy, brilliant audiotapes and a workbook, *Working with Your Shadow*. P. O. Box 691867, Orlando, Florida 32869-1867, 1997.

Cooper, R. C. *Health and Fitness Excellence*. Boston: Houghton Mifflin, 1989.

Eliot, R. S. *From Stress to Strength.* New York: Bantam, 1944.

Hobbs, C. *Stress and Natural Healing.* Loveland, Colorado: Interweave Press, 1997.

Huxley, A. *The Perennial Philosophy.* New York: Harper & Row, 1945.

Jaffe, D. *Healing from Within.* New York: Alfred A. Knopf, 1980.

Jeffers, S. *Feel the Fear and Do It Anyway.* New York: Harcourt Brace Jovanovich, 1987.

Lazarus, A. A., and Lazarus, C. N. *The 60-Second Shrink.* San Luis Obispo, Calif.: Impact, 1997.

Moore, T. *Care of the Soul.* New York: HarperCollins, 1992.

Pizzorno, J. *Total Wellness.* Rockin, Calif.: Prima Publishing, 1996.

Sinatra, S. T., *Optimum Health.* New York: Bantam, 1997.

Weil, A. *Health and Healing.* Boston: Houghton Mifflin, 1988.

Weil, A. *Spontaneous Healing.* New York: Alfred A. Knopf, 1995.

APPENDIX B:
ORGANIZATIONS FOR FURTHER
INFORMATION ON HERBS

Herb Research Foundation
1007 Pearl Street, Suite 200
Boulder, CO 80302
phone: (303) 449–2265
fax: (303) 449–7849
www.herbs.org

The Herb Research Foundation (HRF) is a nonprofit organization dedicated to providing accurate and unbiased information on the health benefits of plants. Information services include the Natural Healthcare Hotline for fast answers to questions about using herbs for health, Herb Information Packets on plants and health conditions, and custom botanical literature research. Membership benefits include a complementary subscription to HerbalGram or Herbs for Health magazines, a quarterly newsletter, and discounts on all information services. HRF also provides comprehensive reading lists and other resources for the general public and health care professionals for a nominal fee.

The Natural Healthcare Hotline draws upon a unique database made up of scientific information on more than two hundred plants. Hotline information specialists are trained to offer unbiased answers to questions about herbs and health without diagnosing, prescribing, or recommending specific brands or products. The continuously updated Hotline database contains documented facts on health benefits, safety, known contraindications and drug interactions, and dosage—all the information you need to use herbs correctly to enhance health and well-being.

For more information on joining HRF or to access the Natural Healthcare Hotline, call (303) 449–2265.

American Botanical Council
P.O. Box 201660
Austin, TX 78720
phone: (512) 331–8868
fax: (512) 331–1924
www.herbs.org

The American Botanical Council's main goal is to educate the public about beneficial herbs and plants. This nonprofit organization serves to disseminate accurate scientific information on herbs and herbal research; increase public awareness and professional knowledge of the historic role and current potential of plants in medicine; contribute information to professional and scientific literature that helps establish accurate, credible toxicological and pharmacological data on numerous types of plants and plant materials; promote understanding regarding the importance of preserving native plant populations in temperate and tropical zones; provide the public with original research and reprints of plant-related articles, audio/video tapes, books, and other educational materials; and assist the Herb Research Foundation in achieving its research and educational goals. Germany's Commission E monographs have been translated into English and published by the American Botanical Council.

American Herbal Pharmacopoeia
P.O. Box 5159
Santa Cruz, CA 95063
phone: (408) 438-1700
fax: (408) 461-6317

The American Herbal Pharmacopoeia is a non-profit foundation dedicated to the development of producing monographs containing information about the qualitative and therapeutic characteristics of herbal medicines. The inherent value of herbal medicine in health care necessitates the development of authoritative, critically-reviewed monographs. Presently, in the United States, such information is lacking.

These peer-reviewed monographs will provide health professionals, consumers, manufacturers, and regulatory agencies with essential information on the safe and effective use of botanicals. They will also provide manufacturers with information that will help in every aspect of quality control to assure that herbal products are manufactured in a way that assures the highest degree of safety and effectiveness.

The AHP has a goal of issuing monographs on approximately 300 botanicals including Ayurvedic, Chinese and Western herbs that are commonly used in America. To accomplish this, committees have been established to work collectively in developing various sections of the monographs. In addition, a review committee of experts in the field of herbal medicine has been convened to review the material put togethr by each committee. The committees consist of botanists, herbalists, pharmacists, pharmacognosists, pharmacologists, physicians, and analytical chemists, as well as specialists in Ayurvedic, Chinese and Western herbal medicine.

The goal of the AHP is for each monograph to have the highest degree of accuracy, comprehensiveness, and credibility as is attainable. AHP is collaborating with experts and academic institutions in the United States and abroad to accomplish this.

APPENDIX C:
HERBAL MEDICINE
PRACTITIONERS AND RESOURCES

The following organizations can provide you with information on their specific fields of expertise and assist you in finding herbal medicine practitioners in your area.

Alliance for Alternative
  Medicine
160 N.W. Widmer Place
Albany, OR 97321
phone: (503) 926–4678

American Academy of
  Osteopathy
3500 De Pauw Boulevard,
  Suite 1080
Indianapolis, IN 46268
phone: (317) 879–1881

American Association of
  Acupuncture and Oriental
  Medicine
433 Front Street
Catasauqua, PA 18032
phone: (610) 266–1433
fax: (610) 264–2768
e-mail: AAOM1@AOC.com

*Send $5.00 for a list of members in
any three states.*

American Association of
  Naturopathic Physicians
601 Valley Street, #105
Seattle, WA 98109
phone: (206) 298–0126
fax: (206) 298–1029

*Written requests only. Send $5.00 for
a list of practitioners.*

American Chiropractic
  Association
1701 Clarendon Boulevard
Arlington, VA 22209
phone: (703) 276–8800

American Foundation
  for Alternative Health
  Care
25 Landfield Avenue
Monticello, NY 12701
phone: (914) 794–8181

American College for
Advancement in Medicine
23121 Verdugo Drive, Suite 204
Laguna Hills, CA 92653
phone: (800) 532-3688

American Foundation of
Traditional Chinese
Medicine
505 Beach Street
San Francisco, CA 94133
phone: (415) 776-0502

American Herbalists Guild
P.O. Box 746555
Arvada, CO 80006
phone: (303) 423-8800
fax: (303) 423-8828
www.healthy.com/herbalists

*Written requests only. Send $7.95 for a
list of practitioners.*

American Holistic Medical
Association and American
Holistic Nurses Association
4101 Lake Boone Trail, Suite 201
Raleigh, NC 27607
phone: (919) 787-5146

*Written requests only. Send $8.00 for a
directory of members, all of whom are
either M.D.'s, D.O.'s (osteopaths), or
R.N.'s.*

American Osteopathic
Association
142 E. Ontario Street
Chicago, IL 60611
phone: (312) 280-5800

American Society for
Phytotherapy
P.O. Box 3679
South Pasadena, CA 91031
phone: (818) 457-1742

Aromatherapy Institute of
Research
P.O. Box 2354
Fair Oaks, CA 95628
phone: (916) 965-7546

Association for Network
Chiropractic
P.O. Box 147
Yonkers, NY 10710
phone: (718) 891-4077

Association of Health
Practitioners
P.O. Box 5007
Durango, CO 81301
phone: (303) 259-1091

Ayurveda Institute
P.O. Box 23445
Albuqueruqe, NM 87192-1445

Bach Centre
P.O. Box 320
Woodmere, NY 11598
phone: (516) 825-2229

The Chopra Center for
Well Being
7630 Fay Avenue
La Jolla, CA 92037
phone: (619) 551-7788; (888)
424-6772 (toll free)

Ellon Bach, U.S.A., Inc.
644 Merrick Road
Lynbrook, NY 11563
phone: (516) 593–2206

Homeopathic Association of
    Naturopathic Physicians
14653 Graves Road
Mulino, OR 97042
phone: (503) 829–7326

Institute for Traditional
    Medicine
2017 S.E. Hawthorne
Portland, OR 97214
(no phone calls)

International Association of
    Holistic Health Practitioners
3419 Thom Boulevard
Las Vegas, NV 89106
phone: (702) 873–4542

International Chiropractic
    Association
1110 North Glebe Road,
    Suite 1000
Arlington, VA 22201
phone: (703) 528–5000

Maharishi Ayur-Veda
Maharishi Ayurvedic
    Association of America
P.O. Box 282
Fairfield, IA 52556
phone: (515) 472–8477

National Center for
    Homeopathy
801 North Fairfax Street,
    Suite 306
Alexandria, VA 22314
phone: (703) 548–7790

*Send $7.00 for a list of practitioners,
pharmacies, and other resources.*

National College of
    Naturopathic Medicine
11231 S.E. Market Street
Portland, OR 97216
phone: (503) 255–4860

National Directory of
    Chiropractic
P.O. Box 10056
Olathe, KS 66051
phone: (800) 888–7914

Physicians Committee for
    Responsible Medicine
P.O. Box 6322
Washington, DC 20015
phone: (202) 686–2210

World Chiropractic Alliance
2950 N. Dobson Road, Suite 1
Chandler, AZ 85224
phone: (602) 786–9235/(800)
    347–1011

APPENDIX D:
NATIONAL ASSOCIATIONS
OF MENTAL HEALTH
PROFESSIONALS

American Psychiatric
Association
1400 K Street, NW
Washington, DC 20005
phone: (202) 682–6142

Callers are referred to the local district office in the caller's area, where they will talk with a psychiatrist. The nature of each caller's problem is assessed, and a referral is then made to one or more practitioners who have experience with the caller's problem or issue.

American Psychological
Association
1200 17th Street, NW
Washington, DC 20036
phone: (202) 336–5500

Callers are referred to the state branch office, where the caller's name and number are taken. A referral coordinator returns the call and can provide a list of qualified psychologists and mental health centers in the caller's local area.

Association for the
Advancement of Behavior
Therapy
305 Seventh Avenue
New York, NY 10001
phone: (212) 647–1890

Cognitive Dynamic Therapy
Associates
201 N. Craig Street, Suite 408
Pittsburgh, PA 15213
phone: (412) 687–8700

A referral coordinator can provide a list of qualified cognitive therapists in the caller's local area.

Multi-modal Behavior Therapy
Institute
330 North Harrison Street,
Suite 1A
Princeton, NJ 08540
phone: (609) 683–9122

A referral can be obtained to qualified behavior therapists trained by the founder of multi-modal behavior therapy, Arnold A. Lazarus, Ph.D.

National Association of
   Cognitive-Behavioral
   Therapists
phone: (800) 853–1135
www.nacbt.org.

National Association of Social
   Workers
7981 Eastern Avenue
Silver Spring, MD 20910
phone: (202) 408–8600

The association provides callers with
the names of members in its Clinical
Registry and makes referrals to mem-
bers in the caller's local area.

APPENDIX E:
ANXIETY SELF-HELP GROUPS

Agoraphobics in Motion (AIM)
1729 Crooks Street
Royal Oak, MI 48067–1306
phone: (248) 547–0400

Provides a hotline, newsletter, and list of support groups for anxiety disorders.

Alcoholics Anonymous
P.O. Box 459
Grand Central Station
New York, NY 10163
phone: (212) 870–3400

The original 12-step program, for alcohol abuse.

Anxiety Disorders Association
of America
6000 Executive Boulevard,
Suite 513
Rockville, MD 20852
phone: (301) 231–9350

Provides lists of mental health professionals specializing in the treatment of anxiety disorders and the self-help groups in your area. Offers a newsletter, catalog of books and brochures, and an annual national conference.

Chronic Fatigue Syndrome
Survival Association
P.O. Box 1889
Davis, CA 95617
phone: (916) 756–9242

Patient contacts, referrals to support groups, and access to other resources.

Emotional Anonymous
P.O. Box 4245
St. Paul, MN 55204
phone: (612) 647–9712

A 12-step program for emotional problems.

Freedom from Fear
308 Seaview Avenue
Staten Island, NY 10305
phone: (718) 351-1717

Provides a newsletter on anxiety research and treatments and a support network.

National Alliance for the
    Mentally Ill
200 N. Globe Road, Suite 1015
Arlington, VA 22203–3754
phone: (800) 950–6264

*Provides lists of mental health profes-
sionals and self-help groups for mental
illness in your area.*

National Anxiety Foundation
3135 Custer Drive
Lexington, KY 40517
phone: (606) 272–7166

*Provides referrals to mental health
professionals, resources, and information about self-help groups.*

National Depressive and Manic-
    Depressive Association
730 N. Franklin Street,
    Suite 501
Chicago, IL 60619
phone: (800) 826–3632
fax: (312) 642–7243

*Self-help groups for depression and
manic-depression.*

National Foundation for
    Depressive Illness
P.O. Box 2257
New York, NY 10116–2257
phone: (800) 248–4344

Self-help groups for depression.

National Institute of Mental
    Health
Panic/Anxiety Disorder
    Education Program
Room 7C–02
5600 Fishers Lane
Rockville, MD 20857
phone: (800) 64-PANIC

*Call for a list of books, information,
and resources about panic disorder.*

National Mental Health
    Association
1021 Prince Street
Alexandria, VA 22311–2971
phone: (703) 684–7722; (800)
    969-NMHA

*Provides a list of mental health orga-
nizations, community clinics, and self-
help groups in your area.*

National Organization for
    Victim Assistance (NOVA)
1757 Park Road, NW
Washington, DC 20012
phone: (800) TRY-NOVA

*A private, nonprofit organization that
provides information and referrals for
victims of crime.*

National Victim Center
2111 Wilson Boulevard,
    Suite 300
Arlington, VA 22201
phone: (800) 394–2255

*Offers a toll-free information line with
access to more than five thousand vic-
tim-assistance programs nationwide.*

Nicotine Anonymous
P.O. Box 591777
San Francisco, CA 94159—1777
phone: (415) 750—0328

A 12-step program for nicotine addiction.

Obsessive Compulsive Disorder
Foundation
P.O. Box 70
Milford CT 06460
(203) 878—5669; (203)
874—3843 is a 24-hour
information line

Offers books, brochures, and video-tapes. A bimonthly newsletter goes to people with the disorder and their families who become members.

Obsessive Compulsives
Anonymous
P.O. Box 215
New Hyde Park, NY 11040
phone: (516) 741—4901

A 12-step program to support persons with obsessive-compulsive disorder and their families.

Phobics Anonymous
P.O. Box 1180
Palm Springs, CA 92263
phone: (760) 322-COPE

A 12-step program to support persons with anxiety disorders and their families.

Recovery, Inc.
802 N. Dearborn Street
Chicago, IL 60610
phone: (312) 337—5661

Self-help groups for anxiety and other mental health disorders.

APPENDIX F:
INTERNET RESOURCES
FOR ANXIETY AND HERBS

Attention Deficit Hyperactivity
   Disorder Page
http://www.healthguide.com/ADHD

Algy's Home Page—Medicinal
http://www.algy.com/herb/

American Botanical Council
http://www.herbalgram.org./
   abcmission.html

American Herbalists Guild
http://www.healthy.com/herbalists

American Mental Health Alliance
http://www.psych.org

Ask Dr. Weil
http://www.drweil.com

Health World
http://www.healthworld.com/

Henrietta's Herbal Homepage
http://www.sunsite.unc.edu/
   herbmed/

Herbal Blessings
http://www.herbalblessings.com

Herbal Hall
http://www.herb.com/herbal.htm

Herb Research Foundation
http://www.herbs.org

Hypericum
http://www.hypericum.com

Mental Health
http://www.mentalhealth.com/

Mental Health Net
httpp://www.cmhc.com/

National Institute of Mental
   Health
http://www.nimh.nih.gov

Obsessive Compulsive Disorder
   Foundation
http://www.pages.prodigy.com/
   alwillen/ocf.html

Office of Alternative Medicine
http://altmed.od.nih.gov.

Office of Dietary Supplements
http://dietary-
   supplements.info.nih.gov.

Stress Release
http://www.stressrelease.com/
   strssbus.html

NOTES

CHAPTER 5

1. Adapted from American Psychiatric Association, *The Diagnostic and Statistical Manual of Mental Disorders*, ed. 4 (Washington, D.C.: APA, 1994).

CHAPTER 8

1. G. E. Valliant, *Adaptation to Life* (Boston: Little Brown, 1977).

CHAPTER 9

1. David Eisenberg et al, "Unconventional Medicine in the United States," *New England Journal of Medicine* (January 28, 1993): 246–252.

CHAPTER 10

1. There are other means to create that consistency besides standardization, however. Many herbal remedies use a potency ratio that tells how much of the product is equal to a given amount of herb. For example, a potency ratio of 4:1 means that the product is four times as concentrated as the herb itself. This system is frequently used for liquid extracts.

CHAPTER 11

1. R. F. Weiss, *What Is Herbal Medicine?* (Beaconsfield, England: Beaconsfield Publishers, 1988).

CHAPTER 13

1. Please see Harold H. Bloomfield, M.D., Mikael Nordfors, M.D., and Peter McWilliams, *Hypericum and Depression* (Los Angeles: Prelude Press, 1996).

CHAPTER 14

1. C. Wolfman, H. Viola, A. Paladini et al, "Possible anxiolytic effects of chrysin, a central benzodiazepine receptor ligand isolated from Passiflora coerulea," *Pharmacology, Biochemistry and Behavior* 47 (1994):1−4.

CHAPTER 22

1. Please see Harold H. Bloomfield, M.D., with Leonard Felder, Ph.D., *Making Peace with Yourself* (New York: Ballantine, 1985).

CHAPTER 23

1. Please see Harold H. Bloomfield, M.D., and Robert K. Cooper, Ph.D., *The Power of 5* (Emmaus, Pa.: Rodale, 1995).
2. *Journal of the American Medical Association* 276 (1996): 1473−1479.
3. *Medical Tribune* 14, February 10, 1994.
4. *Journal of the American Medical Association* 274 (1995): 894−901.
5. *American Journal of Managed Care* 3 (1997): 135−144.

CHAPTER 24

1. G. Hendricks and K. Hendricks, "Effects of Daily Breathing on Tiredness and Tension," *At the Speed of Life* (New York: Bantam, 1994), 195−196.
2. *American Heritage Dictionary* (Boston: Houghton Mifflin, 1992).
3. Please see Harold H. Bloomfield and Robert K. Cooper, *How to be Safe in an Unsafe World* (New York: Crown, 1996).
4. K. Eppley, A. Abrams, and J. Shear, "Differential effects of relaxation techniques on trait anxiety: a meta-analysis," *Journal of Clinical Psychology* 45 (1989):957−974.
5. *Psychosomatic Medicine* 49 (1987): 493−505.
6. *Hypertension* 26(5) (1995): 820−827.
7. *American Journal of Managed Care* 4 (1996): 427−437.
8. *American Journal of Health Promotion* 10(3) (1996): 208−216.
9. *Alcoholism Treatment Quarterly* 11 (1994): 41−84.

CHAPTER 27

1. Please see Harold H. Bloomfield, M.D., and Sirah Vettese, Ph.D., with Robert B. Kory, *Lifemates* (New York: Signet, 1992).

CHAPTER 28

1. Please also be sure to read a previous book I co-authored, *How to Survive the Loss of a Love* (Prelude Press, 1976, revised edition 1991), the number one selling guide for coping with loss, and the grief manual most recommended by psychologists to their patients for over twenty years.
2. Please see Harold H. Bloomfield, M.D., with Leonard Felder, Ph.D., *Making Peace with Your Parents* (New York: Ballantine, 1983).
3. Hoffman Quadrinity Process, 223 San Anselmo, CA 94960; (800) 506–5253.

CHAPTER 29

1. For excellent audiotapes and a workbook—*Making Peace with Your Shadow* (Orlando, Florida: Concept Synergy, 1997)— please call (800) 678-2356.

ACKNOWLEDGMENTS

My deepest gratitude to my wife, Sirah Vettese, for her radiant love, total support, and creative input. Her intelligence, wisdom, and compassion shine throughout. Heartfelt appreciation to our children, Shazara, Damien, and Michael, whose work contributed to this book. Much love to my mother, Fridl, departed father, Max, sister, Nora, and brother-in-law, Gus.

Dr. Robert Cooper, a brilliant researcher and writer, contributed mightily and unselfishly to the natural self-healing section. He is my brother in spirit and a great teacher. My heartfelt gratitude to Robert for his unwavering personal and professional support.

Special thanks to Peter McWilliams for the best-selling books we did together at Prelude Press and to Ed Haisha for his excellent promotion of those books. I wish to acknowledge Robert Kory and Leonard Felder for their contributions to my work and life. My heartfelt appreciation to Dr. Mikael Nordfors for his friendship and for his research on *Hypericum*.

My gratitude to Maggie Adams (my devoted typist) and her assistants Charles Adams, Rebekka Adams, and Judy McGrath (manuscript proofreaders). My assistant, Lisa Cardoza, has been invaluable. Heartfelt appreciation to Truen Bergen, Barbara Bourdette, Deepak and Rita Chopra, Bobby Colomby, Ken and Karen Druck, Mike and Donna Fletcher, Trudy Green, Louise Hay, Christopher Hills, Raz and Liza Ingrasci, Noel Johanson (my massage therapist), Mark Laponte (my trainer), Norman and Lyn Lear, Michael Moore, Dan, Dana, and Leah Plant, Jach Pursel, Vince and Laura Regalbuto, Bob Roth, and Ayman and Rowan Sawaf. Special gratitude to Maharishi Mahesh Yogi and Lazaris.

I feel privileged to have the best editor in the whole world, Joelle Delbourgo, Senior Vice President, Associate Publisher, and

Editor-in-Chief of HarperCollins Publishers. I am especially grateful for her commitment to the highest vision for this book, and for her friendship. I also wish to acknowledge the exceptional efforts of Tim Duggan, Joelle's superb assistant. I wish to thank Margret McBride for her enthusiasm, guidance, and continuous support.

My appreciation to Stephanie Lehrer of HarperCollins, Sue Taggart of Adinfinitum, and Larry Zoeller of Selz/Seabolt Communications for their anticipated brilliant public relations efforts.

I am especially grateful to Rob McCaleb, Executive Director of the Herb Research Foundation, and his staff, for helping to provide reliable information on herbs. My thanks to Mark Blumenthal, Donald Brown, Jean Carper, James Duke, Steven Foster, Christopher Hobbs, David Hoffman, Terry Lemerond, Michael Murray, Varro Tyler, Roy Upton, Andrew Weil, and the researchers of herbal medicines worldwide for paving the way. Appreciation goes to Michael Loes and Michael Janson for their expert review of the manuscript.

My respect and admiration goes to John Hagelin, Mike Tompkins, and all the candidates and supporters of the Natural Law Party for serving as champions of natural medicines and preventive health care in their blueprint for a healthy, prosperous America.

BIBLIOGRAPHY

Allain, H., Raoul, P., Lieury, A. et al. Effect of two doses of Ginkgo biloba extract (EGb 761) on the dual-coding test in elderly subjects. *Clinical Therapy* 15:549–558, 1993.

Armanini, D. Further studies on the mechanism of the mineralocorticoid action of licorice in humans. *Journal of Endocrinological Investigation* 19(9):624–629, 1996.

Ashton, C., Whitworth, G., Seldomridge, J. et al. Self-hypnosis reduces anxiety following coronary artery bypass surgery: a prospective, randomized trial. *Journal of Cardiovascular Surgery* 38(1):69–75, 1997.

Awang, D. Milk thistle. *Current Therapeutic Research* 53:533–545, 1993.

Balderer, G., and Borbely, A. Effect of valerian on human sleep. *Psychopharmacology* 87:406–409, 1985.

Baschetti, R. Chronic fatigue syndrome and neurally mediated hypotension. *Journal of the American Medical Association* 275:359, 1996.

Bergner, P. Ginseng: short term effects. *Medical Herbalism* 2(3):5, 1990.

Bhattacharya, S. et al. Anti-stress activity of sitoindosides VII and VIII, new acylsterylglucosides from Withania somnifera. *Phytotherapy Research* 1(1):32–37, 1987.

———. Anxiolytic activity of Panax ginseng roots: an experimental study. *Journal of Ethnopharmacology* 34:87–92, 1991.

Blumenthal, M., ed. *The German Commission E Monographs*. Austin, Tex.: American Botanical Council, 1997.

Bone, K. Kava: a safe herbal treatment for anxiety. *Townsend Letter for Doctors*, June 1995, 84–88.

Borst, J.G.G. Synergistic action of licorice and cortisone in Addison's and Simmonds' disease. *Lancet* 1:657–663, 1953.

Bou-Holaigah, I. The relationship between neurally mediated

hypotension and the chronic fatigue syndrome. *Journal of the American Medical Association* 274:961–967, 1995.

Bradley, P., ed. *British Herbal Compendium.* Vol. 1. British Herbal Medicine Association, 1992.

Brinker, F. *Eclectic Dispensatory of Botanical Therapeutics.* Vol. 2. Eclectic Medical Publications, 1995.

Brown, D. J. *Herbal Prescriptions for Better Health.* Rocklin, California: Prima Publishing, 1996.

Buzzelli, G. A pilot study on the liver protective effect of silybin-phosphatidylcholine complex (IdB1016) in chronic active hepatitis. *International Journal of Clinical Pharmacology and Therapeutic Toxicology* 31:456–460, 1993.

Cai, L. J. et al. Influence of ginseng saponin on the circadian rhythm of brain monoamine neurotransmitters. In *Chronobiology: Its Role in Clinical Medicine, General Biology and Agriculture,* Part B:135–144. New York: Wiley-Liss, 1990.

Carper, J. *Miracle Cures.* New York: HarperCollins, 1997.

Carrescia, O., Benelli, L., Saraceni, F. et al. Silymarin in the prevention of hepatic damage by psychopharmacologic drugs: experimental premises and clinical evaluations. *Clinica Terapeutica* 95:157–164, 1980.

Chang, H., and But, P., eds. *Pharmacology and Applications of Chinese Materia Medica.* World Scientific, 1986.

Cleare, A. J. Contrasting neuroendocrine responses in depression and chronic fatigue syndrome. *Journal of Affective Disorders* 35:283–289, 1995.

Colquhoun, I., and Bunday, S. Lack of essential fatty acids as a possible cause of hyperactivity in children. *Medical Hypotheses* 7:673–679, 1981.

Cummings, S., and Ullman, D. *Everybody's Guide to Homeopathic Medicines.* New York: Putnam, 1991.

D'Angelo, L. et al. A double-blind, placebo-controlled clinical study on the effect of a standardized ginseng extract on psychomotor performance in healthy volunteers. *Journal of Ethnopharmacology* 16:15–22, 1986.

Davies, L. et al. Effects of kava on benzodiazepine and GABA receptor binding. *European Journal of Pharmacology* 183:558, 1990.

Demitrack, M. A. Evidence for impaired activation of the hypothal-amic-pituitary-adrenal axis in patients with chronic fatigue syndrome. *Journal of Clinical Endrocrinology and Metabolism* 73:1224–1234, 1991.

DeSmet, P. A. G. M., ed. *Adverse Effects of Herbal Drugs*. New York: Springer-Verlag, 1993.

Dorling, E. et al. Do ginsenosides influence performance? Results of a double blind study. *Notabene Medici* 10(5):241–246, 1980. (English translation produced by Ginsana.)

Duke, J. A. *The Green Pharmacy*. Emmaus, Pa.: Rodale Press, 1997.

Dunn, C. et al. Sensing an improvement: an experimental study to evaluate the use of aromatherapy, massage and periods of rest in an intensive care unit. *Journal of Advanced Nursing* 21:34–40, 1995.

Farnsworth, N. R. et al. Siberian ginseng: current status as an adaptogen. In *Economic and Medicinal Plant Research*, edited by H. Wagner and N. Farnsworth. Vol. 1. New York: Academic Press, 1985.

Feher, J., Deak, G. et al. Liver protective action of silymarin therapy in chronic alcoholic liver diseases. *Orvosi Hetilap* 130(51):2723–2727, 1989.

Ferenci, R. Randomized controlled trial of silymarin treatment in patients with cirrhosis of the liver. *Journal of Hepatology* 9:105–113, 1989.

Fintelmann, A. The therapeutic activity of Legalon in toxic hepatic disorders demonstrated in a double blind trial. *Therapiewoche* 30:5589–5594, 1980.

Foster, S. *Herbs for Your Health*. Loveland, Colo.: Interweave Press, 1996.

Fritz-Weiss, R. *Herbal Medicine*. AB Arcanum, 1988.

Fulder, S. et al. A double-blind clinical trial of Panax ginseng in aged subjects. In *Proceedings of the 4th International Ginseng Symposium*. Korea Ginseng and Tobacco Research Institute, 1984.

———. Ginseng and the hypothalmic-pituitary control of stress. *American Journal of Chinese Medicine* 9(2):112–118, 1981.

Gengtao, L. et al. Some pharmacological actions of the spores of Ganoderma lucidum and the mycelium of Ganoderma capense cultivated by submerged fermentation. *Chinese Medical Journal* 92(7):495–500, 1979.

Ghosal, S. et al. Immunomodulatory and CNS effects of sitoindosides IX and X, two new glycowithanolides from Withania somnifera. *Phytotherapy Research* 3(5):201–206, 1989.

Gleitz, J. et al. Kavain inhibits non-stereospecifically veratridine-activated Na+ channels. *Planta Medica* 62:1133–1138, 1996.

———. (+)-Kavain inhibits veratridine-activated voltage-dependent Na+-channels in synaptosomes prepared from rat cerebral cortex. *Neuropharmacology* 34(9):1133–1138, 1995.

Gottlieb, B., ed. *New Choices in Natural Healing.* Emmaus, Pa.: Rodale Press, 1995.

Gould, L. et al. Cardiac effects of chamomile tea. *Journal of Clinical Pharmacology* 13 (11/12):475–479, 1973.

Grandhi, A. et al. A comparative pharmacological investigation of ashwaganda and ginseng. *Journal of Ethnopharmacology* 44:131–135, 1994.

Granger, I. et al. Benzophenanthridine alkaloids isolated from Eschscholtzia californica cell suspension cultures interact with vasopressin (V1) receptors. *Planta Medica* 58:35–38, 1992.

Grassel, E. Effect of Ginkgo-biloba extract on mental performance: double-blind study using computerized measurement conditions in patients with cerebral insufficiency. *Fortschritte der Medizin* 110:73–76, 1992.

Green, M., and Keville, K. *Aromatherapy: A Complete Guide to the Healing Art.* Freedom, Calif.: Crossing Press, 1995.

Hallstrom, C. et al. Effects of ginseng on the performance of nurses on night duty. *Comparative Medicine East and West* 6(4):277–282, 1982.

Halstead, B., and Hood, L. *Eleutherococcus senticosus: Siberian Ginseng: An Introduction to the Concept of Adaptogenic Medicine.* Oriental Healing Arts Institute, 1984.

Heinze, H. et al. Pharmacological effects of oxazepam and kava extract in a visual search paradigm assessed with event-related potentials. *Pharmacopsychiatry* 27:224–230, 1994.

Hendricks, H. et al. Central nervous depressant activity of valerenic acid in the mouse. *Planta Medica* 51:28–31, 1985.

Hiai, S. et al. Stimulation of pituitary-adrenocortical system by ginseng saponin. *Endocrinologia Japonica* 26:661–665, 1979.

Hobbs, C. *The Ginsengs.* Santa Cruz, Calif.: Botanica Press, 1996.

———. *Handbook for Herbal Healing: A Concise Guide to Herbal Products.* Santa Cruz, Calif.: Botanica Press, 1994.

———. *Medicinal Mushrooms.* Santa Cruz, Calif.: Botanica Press, 1995.

———. *Stress and Natural Healing.* Loveland, Colo.: Interweave Press, 1997.

———. *Valerian: The Relaxing and Sleep Herb.* Santa Cruz, Calif.: Botanica Press, 1993.

Hofferberth, B. The efficacy of Egb 761 in patients with senile dementia of the Alzheimer type, a double-blind, placebo-controlled study on different levels of investigation. *Human Psychopharmacology* 9:215–222, 1994.

Hoffman, D. *An Herbal Guide to Stress Relief.* Rochester, Vt.: Healing Arts Press, 1991.

Hoffmann, F., Beck, C., Schutz, A., and Offermann, P. Ginkgo extract (Egb 761) (tenobin)/HAES versus naftidrofuryl (Dusodril)/HAES: a randomized study of therapy of sudden deafness. *Laryngorhinootologie* 73:149–152, 1994.

Hong, S., and Koo, J. The effect of the saponin fraction of Panax ginseng on the antioxidant activity of tocopherol. In *Proceedings of the 4th International Ginseng Symposium.* Korean Ginseng and Tobacco Research Institute, 1984.

Hoyer, S. Possibilities and limits of therapy of cognition disorders in the elderly. *Zeitschrift fur Gerontologie Geriatrie* 28(6):457–62, 1995.

Hsu, H. *Oriental Materia Medica.* OHAI Press, 1986.

Hubner, W. et al. Hypericum treatment of mild depression with somatic symptoms. *Journal of Geriatric Psychiatry and Neurology* 7 (suppl 1):S12–14, 1994.

Huguet, F. Decreased cerebral 5-HTIA receptors during aging: reversal by ginkgo biloba extract (Egb 761). *Journal of Pharmacy and Pharmacology* 46:316–318, 1994.

Itil, T. Early diagnosis and treatment of memory disturbances. *American Journal of Electromedicine* (June):81–85, 1996.

————. Natural substances in psychiatry—ginko biloba in dementia. *Psychopharmacology Bulletin* 31:147–158, 1995.

Jones, K. Reishi (Ganoderma): longevity herb of the Orient (Part I). *Townsend Letter for Doctors*, October 1992, 814–818.

————. Reishi (Ganoderma): longevity herb of the Orient (Part II). *Townsend Letter for Doctors*, November 1992, 1008–1012.

Jossofie, A. et al. Kavapyrone enriched extract from Piper methysticum as modulator of the GABA binding site in different regions of rat brain. *Psychopharmacology* 116:469–474, 1994.

Kaminsky, P., and Katz, R. *Flower Essence Repertory: A Comprehensive Guide to North American and English Flower Essences for Emotional and Spiritual Well-Being.* Nevada City, Calif.: Flower Essence Society, 1994.

Kanowski, S. et al. Proof of efficacy of the Ginkgo biloba special extract Egb 761 in outpatients suffering from mild to moderate primary degenerative dementia of the Alzheimer type or multi-infarct dementia. *Pharmacopsychiatry* 29:47–56, 1996.

Kasahara, Y., and Hikino, H. Central actions of adenosine, a nucleotide of Ganoderma lucidum. *Phytotherapy Research* 1(4):173–176, 1987.

————. Central actions of Ganoderma lucidum. *Phytotherapy Research* 1(1):17–21, 1987.

Keung, W. M. Daidzin and daidzein suppress free choice ethanol intake by Syrian golden hamsters. *Proceedings of the National Academy of Sciences* 90:10008–10012, 1993.

Kleijnen, J. Ginkgo biloba for cerebral insufficiency. *British Journal of Clinical Pharmacology* 34(4):352–358, 1992.

Kohnen, R., and Oswald, W. D. The effects of valerian, propranolol and their combination on activation, performance and mood of healthy volunteers under social stress conditions. *Pharmacopsychiatry* 21:447–448, 1988.

Koltringer, P., Langsteger, W., Klima, G., Reisecker, F., and Eber, O. Hemorheologic effects of ginkgo biloba extract Egb 761: dose-dependent effect of Egb 761 on microcirculation and viscoelasticity of blood. *Fortschritte der Medizin* 111:170–172, 1993.

Kunkel, H. EEG profile of three different extractions of Ginkgo biloba. *Neuropsychobiology* 27:40–45, 1993.

Kuppurajan, K. et al. Effect of ashwaganda (Withania somnifera Dunal) on the process of aging in human volunteers. *Journal of Research in Ayurveda and Sidha* 1(1):247–258, 1980.

Leathwood, P. et al. Aqueous extract of valerian reduces latency to fall asleep in man. *Planta Medica* 50:144–148, 1985.

————. Aqueous extract of valerian root (Valeriana officinalis L.) improves sleep quality in man. *Pharmacology, Biochemistry and Behavior* 17:65–71, 1982.

————. Quantifying the effects of mild sedatives. *Journal of Psychiatric Research* 17(2):115–122, 1982/83.

LeBars, P.L., Katz, M. M., Berman, N. et al. A placebo-controlled, double-blind, randomized trial of an extract of Ginkgo biloba for dementia. *Journal of the American Medical Association* 278:1327–1332, 1997.

Lee, K. et al. Effects of Humulus lupulus extract on the central nervous system in mice. *Planta Medica* 59 (suppl):691, 1993.

Lee, S. et al. Chronic intake of Panax ginseng extract stabilizes sleep and wakefulness in food-deprived rats. *Neuroscience Letters* 111:217–221, 1990.

Lehmann, E. et al. Efficacy of a special kava extract (Piper methysticum) in patients with states of anxiety, tension and excitedness of non-mental origin: a double-blind placebo-controlled study of four weeks treatment. *Phytomedicine* 3(2):113–119, 1996.

Lieberman, S., and Bruning, N. *The Real Vitamin and Mineral Book.* Avery, 1990.

Lindahl, O., and Lindwall, L. Double-blind study of a valerian preparation. *Pharmacology, Biochemistry and Behavior* 32:1065–1066, 1989.

Linde, K., Clausius, N., Ramirez, G., Eifel, F., Hedges, L., Jonas, W. Are the clinical effects of homeopathy placebo effects? A meta-analysis of placebo-controlled trials. *Lancet* 350:834–843, 1997.

Linde, K., Ramirez, G,. Mulrow, C. D., Pauls, A., Weidenhammer, W., Melchart, D. Saint-John's-wort for depression: an overview and meta-analysis of randomized clinical trials. *British Medical Journal* 313:253–258, 1996.

Lindenberg, V. D., and Pitule-Schodel, H. D,L-kavain in comparison with oxazepam in anxiety states: a double-blind clinical trial. *Deutscher Medizin* 108(2):31–34, 1990.

Low Dog, T. A common sense approach to attention deficit hyperactive disorder. In *Medicines from the Earth: Exploring Nature's Pharmacy. Official Proceedings, Blue Ridge Mountain Assembly 5/31–6/2, 1997.* Gaia Herbal Research Institute, 1997.

Maluf, E. et al. Assessment of the hypnotic/sedative effects and toxicity of Passiflora edulis aqueous extract in rodents and humans. *Phytotherapy Research* 5:262–266, 1991.

Mascarella, S. Therapeutic and antilipoperoxidant effects of silybanphosphatidylcholine complex in chronic liver disease: preliminary results. *Current Therapeutic Research* 53(1):98–102, 1993.

Matthews, J. et al. Effects of the heavy usage of kava on physical health: summary of a pilot survey in an aboriginal community. *Medical Journal of Australia* 148:548–555, 1988.

Medon, P. et al. Effects of Eleutherococcus senticosus extracts on hexobarbital metabolism in vivo and in vitro. *Journal of Ethnopharmacology* 10:235–241, 1984.

Menon, N., and Dhopeshwarkar, G. Essential fatty acid deficiency and brain development. *Progress in Lipid Research* 21:309–326, 1982.

Morazzoni, P., and Bombardelli, E. Valeriana officinalis: traditional use and recent evaluation of activity. *Fitoterapia* 66(2):99–112, 1995.

Mowrey, D. *Herbal Tonic Therapies.* New Canaan, Conn.: Keats Publishing, 1993.

Mueller, W. E., Rolli, M., Schäfer, C., and Hafner, U. Effects of Hypericum extract (LI 160) in biochemical models of antidepressant activity. *Pharmacopsychiatry* 30 (suppl):102–107, 1997.

Munte, T. et al. Effects of oxazepam and an extract of kava roots (Piper methysticum) on event-related potentials in a word recognition task. *Neuropsychobiology* 27:46–53, 1993.

Muriel, P., Garciapina, T., Perez-Alvarez, V., and Mourelle, M. Silymarin protects against paracetamol-induced lipid peroxidation and liver damage. *Journal of Applied Toxicology* 12:439–442, 1992.

Murray, M. The clinical use of Hypericum perforatum. *American Journal of Natural Medicine* 2(3):10–12, 1995.

———. *Encyclopedia of Nutritional Supplements.* Rocklin, Calif.: Prima Publishing, 1996.

———. *Getting Well Naturally Series: Stress, Anxiety and Insomnia.* Rocklin, Calif.: Prima Publishing, 1994.

———. *The Healing Power of Herbs.* 2d ed. Rocklin, Calif.: Prima Publishing, 1995.

———. *Natural Alternatives to Over the Counter and Prescription Drugs.* New York: William Morrow, 1994.

———. *Natural Alternatives to Prozac.* New York: William Morrow, 1996.

Murray, M., and Werbach, M. *Botanical Influences on Illness.* Tarazana, Calif.: Third Line Press, 1994.

Novack, D., Suchman, A., Clark, W., et al. Calibrating the physician: Personal awareness and effective patient care. *Journal of the American Medical Association* 278:502–509, 1997.

Ogletree, R. L., and Fischer, R. *The Top 10 Scientifically Proven Natural Products.* Brandon, Mass.: Natural Source Digest, 1997.

Owen, R. Ginseng: a pharmacological profile. *Drugs of Today* 17(8):343–351, 1981.

Palasciano, G., Portincasa, P., Palmeri, V. et al. The effect of silymarin on plasma levels of malon-dialdehyde in patients receiving long-term treatment with psychotropic drugs. *Current Therapeutic Research* 55:537–545, 1994.

Pearce, P. et al. Panax ginseng and Eleutherococcus senticosus extracts: in vitro studies on binding to steroid receptors. *Endocrinologia Japonica* 29:567–573, 1982.

Pizzorno, J., and Murray, M., eds. *Encyclopedia of Natural Medicine.* Rocklin, Calif.: Prima Publishing, 1991.

———. *A Textbook of Natural Medicine.* John Bastyr College Publications, 1985.

Plath, P., and Olivier, J. Results of combined low-power laser therapy and extracts of Ginkgo biloba in cases of sensorineural hearing loss and tinnitus. *Advances in Oto-rhino-laryngology* 49:101–104, 1995.

Prabhu, Y. M. et al. Neuropharmacological activity of Withania somnifera. *Fitoterapia* 61(3):237–240, 1990.

Qing-Yao, Y., and Min-Ming, W. The effect of Ganoderma lucidum extract against fatigue and endurance in the absence of oxygen. In *Proceedings of Contributed Symposium*, 5th International Mycological Congress, Vancouver, August 14–21, 1994:101–104.

Raabe, A., Raabe, M., and Ihm, P. Therapeutic follow-up using automatic perimetry in chronic cerebroretinal ischemia in elderly patients: prospective double-blind study with graduated dose Ginkgo biloba treatment (Egb 761). *Klinische Monatsblatter fur Augenheilkunde* 199:432–438, 1991.

Rapin, J. R., Lamproglou, I., Drieu, K. et al. Demonstration of the anti-stress activity of an extract of Ginkgo biloba (Egb 761) using a discrimination learning task. *General Pharmacology* 25:1009–1016, 1994.

Rauscher, F., Shaw, G., Ky, K. Music and spatial task performance. *Nature* 356:6–11, 1993.

Rector-Page, L. *Healthy Healing*. Healthy Healing Publications, 1992.

————. *How to Be Your Own Herbal Pharmacist*. Healthy Healing Publications, 1991.

Rolland, A. et al. Behavioral effects of the American traditional plant Eschscholzia californica: sedative and anxiolytic properties. *Planta Medica* 57:212–216, 1991.

Rosenfield, M. et al. Evaluation of the efficacy of a standardized ginseng extract in patients with psychophysical asthenia and neurological disorders. *La Semana Medica* 173(9):148–154, 1989. (English translation by Ginsana.)

Sahelian, R. *Kava*. Green Bay, Wisc.: Impakt Communications, 1997.

Saksena, A. et al. Effect of Withania somnifera and Panax ginseng on dopaminergic receptors in rat brain during stress. *Planta Medica* 55:95, 1989.

Saletu, B. et al. EEG-brain mapping, psychometric and psychophysiological studies on central effects of kavain-A, kava plant derivative. *Human Psychopharmacology* 4:169–190, 1989.

Schiraldi, G. R. *Conquer Anxiety, Worry and Nervous Fatigue*. Ellicott City, Md.: Chevron Publishing, 1997.

Schmidt-Voigt, J. Treatment of nervous sleep disturbances and inner restlessness with a purely herbal sedative. *Therapiewoche* 36:663–667, 1986.

Schulz, H. et al. The effect of valerian extract on sleep polygraphy in poor sleepers: a pilot study. *Pharmacopsychiatry* 27:147–151, 1994.

———. Effects of Hypericum extract on the sleep EEG in older volunteers. *Journal of Geriatric Psychiatry and Neurology* 7 (suppl 1):539–543, 1994.

Seifert, T. Therapeutic effects of valerian in nervous disorders: a field study. *Therapeutikon* 2:94–98, 1988.

Semlitsch, H. V., Anderer, P., Saletu, B., Binder, G. A., and Decker, K. A. Cognitive psychophysiology in nootropic drug research: effects of Ginkgo biloba on event-related potentials (P300) in age-associated memory impairment. *Pharmacopsychiatry* 28:134–142, 1995.

Singh, N. et al. Withania somnifera (ashwaganda) a rejuvenating herbal drug which enhances survival during stress (an adaptogen). *International Journal of Crude Drug Research* 20(1):29–35, 1982.

Singh, Y. N. Effects of kava on neuromuscular transmission and muscle contractility. *Journal of Ethnopharmacology* 7:267–276, 1983.

Soulimani, R. et al. Behavioral effects of Passiflora incarnata L. and its indole alkaloid and flavonoid derivatives and maltol in the mouse. *Journal of Ethnopharmacology* 57:11–20, 1997.

———. Neurotropic action of the hydroalcoholic extract of Melissa officinalis in the mouse. *Planta Medica* 57:105–108, 1991.

Speroni, E., and Minghetti, A. Neuropharmacological activity of extracts from Passiflora incarnata. *Planta Medica* 54:488–491, 1988.

Sprecher, E. Ginseng: miracle drug or phytopharmacon? *Apotheker Journal* 9(5):52–61, 1987.

Strokina, T., and Mukho, T. Autonomic disturbances in neuroses and the degree of recovery from them with Eleutherococcus treatment. *Lek. Sredstva Dal'nego. Vostoka* 7:195–199, 1966. Translation from Farnsworth, N., ed. *Special Report on the Chemical Equivalency and Safety of Siberian Ginseng Liquid Extract* (IMEDEX). University of Illinois, 1979.

319

Strokina, T. *Lek. Sredstva Dal'nago Vostoka* 7(1966):201–211. Translation from N. Farnsworth, ed., *Special Report on the Chemical Equivalency and Safety of Siberian Ginseng Liquid Extract* (IMEDEX). Champaign: University of Illinois, 1979.

Strokina, T. *Zhur. Neuropathol. Psychiatry* 67(1967):903–906. Translation from N. Farnsworth, ed., *Special Report on the Chemical Equivalency and Safety of Siberian Ginseng Liquid Extract* (IMEDEX). Champaign: University of Illinois, 1979.

————. The change in vascular tonus in patients with neurasthenia under the action of Eleutherococcus. *Sb. Nauch. Tr. Vladivostok Med. Inst.* 4:19–22, 1968. Translation from Farnsworth, N., ed. *Special Report on the Chemical Equivalency and Safety of Siberian Ginseng Liquid Extract* (IMEDEX). University of Illinois, 1979.

Sugaya, A. et al. Proliferative effect of ginseng saponin on neurite extension of primary cultured neurons of the rat cerebral cortex. *Journal of Ethnopharmacology* 22:173–181, 1988.

Taillandier, J., Ammar, A., Rabourdin, J. P. et al. Ginkgo biloba extract in the treatment of cerebral disorders due to aging. In *Rokan (Ginkgo biloba): Recent Results in Pharmacology and Clinic*, edited by E. W. Funfgeld. New York: Springer-Verlag, 1988: 291–301.

Tyler, V. *Herbs of Choice.* Binghamton, N.Y.: Haworth Press, 1994.

————. *The Honest Herbal.* 3rd ed. Binghamton, N.Y.: Haworth Press, 1993.

Viola, H. et al. Apigenin, a component of Matricaria recutita flowers, is a central benzodiazepine receptors-ligan with anxiolytic effects. *Planta Medica* 61:213–216, 1995.

Volz, H. P., and Kieser, M. Kava-kava extract WS 1490 versus placebo in anxiety disorders: a randomized placebo-controlled 25-week outpatient trial. *Pharmacopsychiatry* 30:1–5, 1997.

Vorbach, E. U., Arnoldt, K. H., and Heubner, W. D. Efficacy and tolerability of Saint-John's-wort extract LI 160 versus Imipramine in patients with severe depressive episodes according to ICD–10. *Pharmacopsychiatry* 30 (suppl):81–85, 1997.

Warnecke, G. Neurovegetative dystonia in the female climacteric: studies on the clinical efficacy and tolerance of kava extract WS 1490. *Fortschritte der Medizin* 109(4):119–122, 1991.

Watanabe, H. et al. Effect of Panax ginseng on age-related changes in the spontaneous motor activity and dopaminergic nervous system in the rat. *Japanese Journal of Pharmacology* 55:51–56, 1991.

Weil, A. *Health and Healing.* Boston: Houghton Mifflin, 1988.

————. *Spontaneous Healing.* New York: Alfred A. Knopf, 1995.

Weiss, R. F. *What Is Herbal Medicine?* Beaconsfield, England: Beaconsfield Publishers, 1988.

Werbach, M. *Nutritional Influences on Illness.* 2d ed. Tarzana, Calif.: Third Line Press, 1996.

Willard, T. *Textbook of Advanced Herbology.* Alberta, Canada: Wild Rose College of Natural Healing, 1993.

————. *Wild Rose Scientific Herbal.* Alberta, Canada: Wild Rose College of Natural Healing, 1991.

Willis, A., and Smith, D. Dihomo-gamma-linoleic and gamma-linolenic acids in health and disease. In *New Protective Roles for Selected Nutrients.* New York: Alan Liss, 1989.

Winston, D. Eclectic specific condition review: attention deficit disorder (ADD)/attention deficit hyperactivity disorder (ADHD). *Protocol Journal of Botanical Medicine* 2(1):38–39, 1996.

Witte, S., Anadere, I., and Walitza, E. Improvement of hemorheology with Ginkgo biloba extract: decreasing a cardiovascular risk factor. *Fortschritte der Medizin* 110:247–250, 1992.

Wohlfart, R. et al. The sedative-hypnotic principle of hops, pharmacology of 2-methyl–3-buten–2-ol. *Planta Medica* 48:120–123, 1983.

Wolfman, C. H., Paldini, V. A. et al. Possible anxiolytic effects of chrysin, a central benzodiazepine receptor ligand isolated from Passiflora coerulea. *Pharmacology, Biochemistry and Behavior* 47:1–4, 1994.

Wotton, E. Naturopathic specific condition review: attention deficit/hyperactivity disorder. *Protocol Journal of Botanical Medicine* 2(1):29–31, 1996.

Yamanaka, W. et al. Essential fatty acid deficiency in humans. *Progress in Lipid Research* 19:187–215, 1981.

Zhang, H., and Huang, J. Preliminary study of traditional Chinese medicine treatment of minimal brain dysfunction: analysis of

100 cases. *Chung Hsi I Chieh Ho Tsa Chih* 10(5):278–279, 1990. (English abstract only.)

―――. Therapy of brain function disorders in the elderly: proven therapeutic results with Ginkgo biloba extract in degenerative and vascular dementia. Report of a symposium. Munich, 7 December 1990. *Fortschritte der Medizin* 107 (suppl):1–19, 1991.

ABOUT THE AUTHOR

Harold H. Bloomfield, M.D., is the psychiatrist America trusts. Yale-trained, Dr. Bloomfield is a renowned leader in herbal medicine and integrative psychiatry. His recent national bestseller, *Hypericum* (Saint-John's-wort) *& Depression,* was featured on *20/20, Good Morning America,* ABC's *The View, CBS This Morning,* as well as in *Time, Newsweek, People, The New York Times,* and *USA Today.* Dr. Bloomfield has frequently appeared on *Oprah, Sally Jesse Raphael, Larry King, Geraldo, Leeza,* FOX and ABC News specials.

Dr. Bloomfield's first book, *TM-Transcendental Meditation,* was an international bestseller. Two of his other bestsellers, *How to Survive the Loss of a Love* and *How to Heal Depression,* have become self-help classics Dr. Bloomfield has been at the forefront of many important self-help movements worldwide for twenty-five years. His books *Making Peace with Your Parents, Making Peace with Yourself, Lifemates,* and *Making Peace in Your Stepfamily* introduced personal, marital, and family peacemaking to millions of people. Dr. Bloomfield's books have sold more than seven million copies and have been translated into twenty-six languages.

Dr. Bloomfield regularly teaches seminars on herbal medicine to physicians and other health care professionals worldwide. Dr. Bloomfield has received the *Medical Self-Care* magazine Book of the Year Award, the Golden Apple Award for Outstanding Psychological Educator and the American Holistic Health Association's Lifetime Achievement Award. He is an adjunct professor of psychology at the Union Graduate School and a member of the American Psychiatric Association and the San Diego Psychiatric Society.

Dr. Bloomfield is a much admired keynote speaker for public programs, corporate meetings, and professional conferences. He maintains a private practice of integrative psychiatry, psychotherapy, and herbal medicine in Del Mar, California. For additional information on Dr. Bloomfield's lectures, seminars, consultations, and products please contact:

Harold H. Bloomfield, M.D.
1337 Camino Del Mar, Suite E
Del Mar, California 92014
(619) 481–9950 (Office)
(619) 792–2333 (Fax)

Dr. Bloomfield will be on the Fall 1998 ballot as Natural Law Party candidate for Governor of California. The Natural Law Party is America's political voice for natural, preventive health care and natural medicines. The Natural Law Party supports the immediate implementation into U.S. health care of prevention-oriented programs that can dramatically cut health care costs and relieve untold anxiety, pain, and suffering. It is the fastest growing political party in America, garnering more than 2.5 million votes nationwide in the 1996 elections. For more information please contact:

The Natural Law Party
P. O. Box 1900
Fairfield, Iowa 52556
(515) 472–2024 (Office)
(515) 472–2011 (Fax)

INDEX

American ginseng, 102, 105–6
  dosage of, 106
  uses of, 106
  See also Ginseng
American Herbal Pharmacopoeia
  (AHP), 292–93
American Herbal Products
  Association, 64
American Horticultural Therapy
  Association, 173
American Psychiatric
  Association, 27–28
Amphetamines, 38, 40
Amygdala
  alarm center in, 31, 32, 48
  aromatherapy and, 130
  kava and, 81
Anafranil (clomipramine), 41,
  74
Anchoring inner safety, 202–4
Anger, 240–58
  common communication traps
    and, 246–58
  constructive vs. destructive,
    243–44
  healing from loss and, 266–67
  making anger work for you,
    241–42
  mental shielding and, 245–46
  rescript and rehearse with,
    244–45
Antiaging chemicals, 175
Antianxiety treatment. *See*
  Treatment of anxiety
Antibiotics, overuse of, 61
Antidepressants, 73–75
  cost of, 59
  diagnosis of anxiety and, 38

milk thistle and damage from,
  110
side effects of, 74
versus *Hypericum*, 59, 84
Anxiety, 1–54
  causes of, 31–36
  diagnosis of, 37–43
  forms of, 3–4
  journaling to express, 222–23
  number of people suffering
    from, 4–5
  predisposition to, 34
  quizzes on, 5–8
  results of leaving untreated,
    10–11
  stimulus-response patterns
    and, 209–10
  time struggle and, 157–58
  treatment of. *See* Anxiety
    treatment
  use of term, 1
Anxiety-anger traps, 247–58
Anxiety attack. *See* Panic attack
Anxiety disorder
  antidepressants for, 73
  primary types of, 25–27
  serotonin imbalance and, 33
  stress and, 52–53
  use of term, 1
Anxiety treatment
  herbal medicine for, 75–77
  homeopathy for, 137–38
  self-healing program for, 77,
    143–44
Apigenin, 95
Approval, and anxiety, 252–53
Aromatherapy, 125, 129–32, 295
Arsenicum, 137